11/08

1 50
used

To my friend, Elaine!!
sisters on the journey!
Love,
Linda

To Elaine -
Happiness, Health + Wisdom!

Alex Holld
3/20/98

VOICES OF QI

*An Introductory Guide
to Traditional Chinese Medicine*

by
Alex Holland, M.Ac., L.Ac.

NORTHWEST INSTITUTE OF
ACUPUNCTURE & ORIENTAL MEDICINE

First Edition   1997

Library of Congress Catalog Card Number 97-092547

ISBN# 0-9622665-3-1

Voices of Qi
The Introductory Guide to Traditional Chinese Medicine
Written by Alex Holland, M.Ac., L.Ac.
Edited by Julie Zinkus
Book Design & Layout by Lanphear Design
Graphic Assistance by John Hughes
Photographs by Linda Joy Stone
Calligraphy by Shou Chun Ma

Published by
Northwest Institute of Acupuncture & Oriental Medicine
1307 N. 45th Street #300
Seattle, WA 98103 USA

Manufactured in the United States

DEDICATION

To my mother, Dorothy, who gave me the freedom to explore, and to my wife, Linda Joy Stone, who joins me on the exploration to freedom...

Acknowledgments

I wish to express my deep gratitude to my teachers in Chinese medicine, especially Dr. Hoy Ping Yee Chan. I am grateful to Dr. Fred Lanphear and the many individuals at the Northwest Institute of Acupuncture and Oriental Medicine who supported me in a number of ways while I was writing this book. It has been a great honor to work with the Northwest Institute.

I want to thank Bob Lanphear for his natural ability to work within the realms of refined quality, using humor and patience as regular forms of communication.

Many thanks to David Kailin whose editorial craftsmanship added an additional level of clarity and depth to the text.

Appreciation and a heart-felt thanks is extended to Fredde Butterworth, Cathy Travis, Marv Thomas, Janet Tricamo, David Pond, Julie Vosoba, and Julie Zinkus for their assistance in smoothing out a sometimes rough manuscript and offering invaluable input.

I wish to thank Barbara Mitchell for diligence, hard work, and keeping the national perspective alive and updated.

I want to acknowledge Franklyn Bradshaw for her inspiration and wisdom.

I would like to thank James Blair for his insights on Oriental medicine.

And lastly I would like to thank Linda Joy Stone, my wife, colleague, in-house editor, photographer, humorist, earth/heart/soul mate, for letting me use the computer while she was doing acupuncture at our clinic. This book could not have been written without her love, patience, and support.

The Pin Yin Phonetic Alphabet
of Consonants and Vowels

The following table shows pronunciations with approximate English equivalents.

a as in *are*
b as in *be*
c like *ts* in *its*
ch as in *cheese*
d as in *duty*
e as in *her*
f as in *fight*
g as in *go*
h between *h* in *her* and *ch* in *chutzpah*
i like the vowel sound in *seat* or the *i* in *sir*
j as in *jeer*
k as in *kick*
l as in *lost*
m as in *more*
n as in *no*
o like the vowel sound in *law*

p as in *park*
q like the *ch* in *China*
r as in *rain*
s as in *sink*
sh as in *shell*
t as in *ten*
u as in *two*
v used only in foreign words or local dialects
w as in *wit*
x like *sh* in *sheep*
y as in *yes*
z as in *zero*
zh like the *j* in *jug*
ai like *ie* in *tie*
ao like *ow* in *cow*
ei like *ay* in *say*
ie like *ie* in *experience*
ou like *oe* in *toe*

Pin Yin is the official standardized English language equivalent that approximates the sounds of the Chinese language.

Explanatory Note

The traditional medicines of Asia have been introduced to the west through rich, diverse, and ancient heritages. Cultural associations representing this diversity and the resulting acronyms, such as TCM for Traditional Chinese Medicine or OM for Oriental Medicine, are often confusing for those not familiar with the roots of Asian medicine, which had its origins in ancient China. Traditional Chinese Medicine developed and holds the foundational principles that gave rise to all other forms of Asian medicine, except that found in India. Traditional Chinese Medicine also uses specific techniques that differentiate it from the traditional medicines of Japan or Korea, which developed methods appropriate to their cultures. From this later perspective then, Traditional Chinese Medicine may also be viewed as a subcategory of the greater umbrella term "Oriental Medicine," which encompasses all traditional medicines throughout Asia. By way of explanation, I have chosen to use the acronym TCM (Traditional Chinese Medicine) throughout this text in my discussions, explanations, and examples because Traditional Chinese Medicine created the unifying philosophy and principles that define all the traditional medicines of the Orient.

FOREWORD

Voices of Qi is a book for those who want to explore the essence of Oriental medicine in a concise and readable format. It is a guide to the patient who wants to understand and participate more fully in the healing power of this form of medicine. It is a handbook for physicians and other medical professionals who need a basic understanding of how this medicine is practiced as a complementary mode of health care.

The increasing interest and use of acupuncture in the U.S. in the past 25 years has been phenomenal. The field of acupuncture, a primary component of Traditional Chinese Medicine (TCM), is one of the fastest growing forms of health care in the U.S. and is making exciting headway in becoming a vital part of the nation's health care system. It was estimated in 1993 that there were 9 to 12 million patient visits for Chinese medicine across the U.S. Acupuncturists are now licensed or allowed to practice in 35 states including the District of Columbia. Over 7000 acupuncturists have been certified nationally. There are currently 33 colleges of acupuncture and Oriental medicine that are accredited or candidates for accreditation and 12 more that have applied. This incredible growth and acceptance of acupuncture shows every evidence of increasing in the next few years.

During this period of rapid assimilation of Oriental medicine into the U.S. there has been a proliferation of various texts, some translated from the original Chinese. Most of these have been written for practitioners of Oriental medicine. A few have been written for the general public. However, few effectively bridge the gap between eastern and western medicine, addressing the questions raised by western trained physicians and other allied health professionals as well as their patients.

Voices of Qi provides a unique way of discovering the art of traditional Chinese medicine as a "whole systems" approach to health care. Those familiar with western medical traditions will discover that the principles and practices of TCM represent a very different medical paradigm. The TCM concepts, many metaphorical in nature, are concisely explained and then illustrated with case studies. The wide variety of techniques utilized in TCM are briefly described and clearly illustrated. With clear and simple presentation, along with the chapter on visiting a practitioner of TCM, *Voices of Qi* provides a helpful familiarization with this very different approach to medical care. The history, scope of practice, legal and educational structure of the profession, along with other information of a more specific nature, are systematically presented in a series of appendices at the end of the book.

In summary, *Voices of Qi* is a tour guide for those wanting to venture into the Oriental medical culture, providing assistance with the language and protocol which is in striking contrast to conventional western medical culture with which we are familiar.

The tour ends with a glimpse into the future of a World Medicine that results as a synergism from these very different approaches to medicine. The emerging new language of energetic medicine undergirded by scientific exploration is introduced as an invitation to be a fellow-traveler on this pathway towards World Medicine.

Fred Lanphear, Ph.D.

President,

Northwest Institute of Acupuncture & Oriental Medicine

September 30, 1997

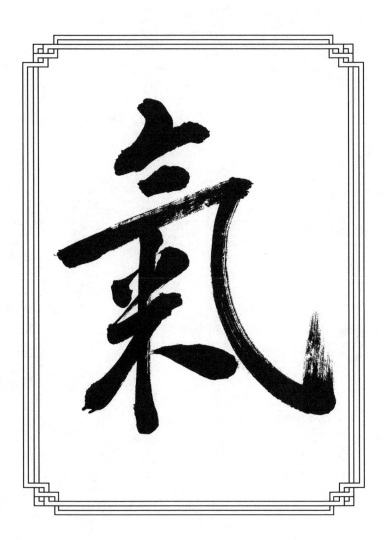

INTRODUCTION

TCM is a complete healing science in and of itself. It has a refined nature and has often been referred to as an art, and to the western mind, its workings remain mostly a mystery. My intention in writing this book is to offer the American public, as well as other health care professionals, a clear presentation of the theory and practice of this ancient medicine. It is evident that its efficacy is being realized, and that this alternative (or complementary) medicine is gaining acceptance in our western health care system. Why are millions drawn to Oriental medicine? How does it work? What are its theories? What can it treat?

These basic questions are difficult to answer if we cling to our culture's dominant way of dissecting the world in which we live. The questions are relevant not only to Chinese medicine, but to breakthroughs in western medicine as well. We are equally compelled to ask, "How does the mental imagery used in some cancer therapies* bring about such remarkable results?" and "What is it in the imagery process that transforms human tissue and enhances the immune response?" Is it the power of the mind? The power of the emotions? Is there a common thread linking medical imagery work with TCM? I invite you to look for the answers in the subtle energetic forces that influence the health of the physical body.

A foundational principle of TCM is the concept of Qi (pronounced chee), commonly understood as the biological vitality of living organisms. In Oriental philosophy the concept of Qi is not restricted to living organisms, although it does represent a very specific functional and organizational process within biological systems. Qi is also conceived of as a universal force that moves planets and orchestrates the reactions of subatomic particles—it is the energetic template on which all of existence is fashioned. Within the small window of biological systems, it is the underlying force that cradles our evolution and propels the organization and processes of everyday existence. Additionally, Qi is also the matter on which this force acts. Matter is simply viewed as *condensed* Qi.

* As prescribed in therapies by Drs. Bernie Siegel, Andrew Weil, Norm Shealy, Larry Dossey, etc.

The Chinese character for Qi (氣) is derived from two separate pictographs that together create a more expansive meaning than either used alone. The original meaning of (气) means "vapor," "breath," or "weather" and denotes energy that is rising upward. The lower character (米) symbolizes "rice" that is bursting with vitality and life. These two pictographs form the character for Qi, which in human beings represents vital energy obtained through proper breathing and nutrition.

Voices of Qi lays a foundation for understanding TCM through the rich concept of vital energy—the universal force of Qi. The physical body that we affirm and treat in western medicine is but a small portion of the subject of healing in TCM. In TCM, we are seen not only as flesh and blood, but as energetic beings of thought, emotions, and spiritual aspirations as well. We are simultaneously spirit and matter, and spirit and matter are both simultaneously Qi. The energetic realms create and define a template through which our physical form is fashioned. Our dense physical body is but the final manifestation of a creative process that begins deep within the unseen world of Qi. Qi is the fundamental concept on which TCM is built.

TCM practitioners weave together seemingly unrelated patterns of signs and symptoms uniting intuition with TCM concepts of body dynamics and disease processes. As an art Chinese medicine not only requires refined skills, but also calls forth expanded human awareness and compassion, as does any good painting, poem, or piece of music.

Experience has led me to believe that the art of TCM lies not only in the skill involved in practicing it, but also through the interpretation of the symbolism of the language. Cloaked in metaphor, this is where the mystery of Chinese thought and medicine is revealed and blossoms. Thus interpretation may be the greatest challenge, for written Chinese is itself a living art. Each pictograph, or character, symbolically represents an action, object, or concept. Open to many nuances of interpretation, we might say that Chinese medicine reveals its artfulness when we loosen our grip on the rational, linear mind and open ourselves to the intuitive, creative process.

Voices of Qi was written to help us redefine and reevaluate the full beauty of who we are. It was written with the understanding that the quality of our thoughts and emotions are major determining factors in the health of our physical bodies. This truth alone puts an incredible responsibility on how we think and what we feel. In the words of the contemporary mystic, Carolyn Myss, from her book, *Anatomy of the Spirit* (Harmony Books, 1996):

"All our thoughts...carry emotional, mental, psychological, or spiritual energy [and] produce biological responses that are then stored in our cellular memory. In this way our biographies are woven into our biological systems, gradually, slowly, every day."

The exploration of TCM takes us on a journey into the energetics behind the creation of health and disease. It is an exploration of the language of symbols and patterned relationships. It is a study in the way of Qi.

TABLE OF CONTENTS

Chapter 1

Foundations of Traditional Chinese Medicine

Chapter 2

Theoretical Framework

Chapter 3

Modalities for Treatment

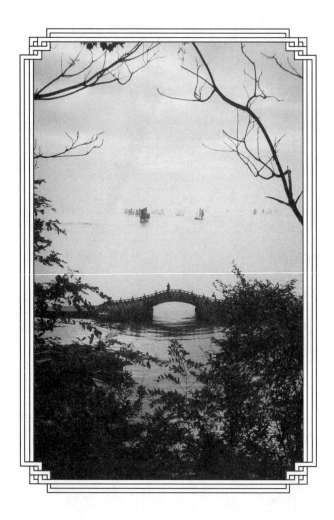

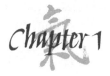

FOUNDATIONS OF TRADITIONAL CHINESE MEDICINE

Understanding the foundations of TCM gives us an appreciation for the way in which this medicine is practiced and the way in which its practitioners view the world. These principles emerged from a cultural heritage steeped in the belief of balance and the unity of all things. The traditional medicine that developed within this cultural framework embraces concepts that, once grasped, lead to a greater appreciation and understanding of our relationship to our world, to each other and to our own health.

BEGINNING

Fundamental to TCM are the powerful roles that balance and harmony play in the role of health. The ancient Chinese observed the cyclical patterns of nature and acknowledged the influences that the starry heavens played in their daily lives. Through patient observation, they realized that all parts of the universe are interrelated. They came to understand our place within nature, recognizing how natural forces strongly influence the affairs of humankind. They understood that we are but a microcosmic reflection of a much greater whole that encompasses all the forces of nature. These forces represent the myriad faces of Qi.

The natural forces of Qi can be broadly divided into the two equal and opposite aspects of Yin and Yang. These Yin and Yang expressions of Qi encompass not only the wilds of nature such as wind, rain, and the cosmic influences of the moon and stars, but also the interpersonal energies at play within our families and communities. The ancient Chinese realized that all of these factors are entwined and contribute to our ability to act and respond to the many situations we encounter daily.

As TCM evolved, these philosophical principles were woven into its foundational fabric. When interpreting these truths within a medical context, it became clear that a well balanced relationship to the world meant living in harmony with all of nature and society, for are we not an integral part of the natural world? The ancient Chinese taught that if we are willing to strive for such a balance, we can fashion a lifestyle that will be reflected in a superior state of health. We will work when it is required and rest as needed. We will eat foods that nourish our bodies and develop healthy relationships with others in our home and workplace. We will listen to our hearts and keep our minds open and strong. The harmonious effect of the Qi of these activities will bring about the healthy integration of our body, mind, spirit, and emotions. The delicate balance will bring order to our lives. We will feel more at peace in the world and more secure in being a part of the larger human community.

BALANCE OF YIN AND YANG

The concepts of Yin and Yang may appear deceptively simple on first appearance, yet they are crucial expressions of the philosophy of balance that has permeated and shaped the cultures of East Asia for thousands of years. The principles of Yin and Yang express all of nature in varying degrees of polarity. They are like two sides of a coin, reflecting complimentary facets of one universal existence. Both are forces of Qi, yet each presents very differently. Yang Qi is the more dynamic, active, male force, symbolically representing the Qi of Heaven. Yin Qi is more foundational, quiescent, and female, symbolically representing the Qi of Earth. According to Chinese philosophy, neither the Yang force nor the Yin force can stand alone, for each must at all times contain at least a small portion of the other equally dynamic force. Yin and Yang symbolically represent the energy of Qi as it manifests in its unlimited and astounding variations.

Traditionally, Yin symbolizes the qualities of Qi found on the dark side of a hill, whereas Yang represents those qualities of Qi found on

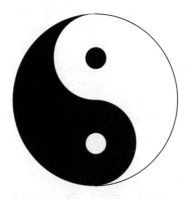

Figure 1: Symbol of Yin and Yang

the sunny side of a hill. The breakdown of the Chinese pictographs for Yin and Yang below expresses this idea more fully:

Yin: 陰   Yang: 陽

阝 represents a hill or mound

云 represents a cloud

日 represents the sun

旦 represents the sun over the horizon

勿 represents rays of light

In addition to those qualities already mentioned, Yang Qi is the component of nature that expresses itself in more active principles such as brightness, expression, daytime, movement, expansion, and so on. Yin Qi, on the other hand, manifests in such qualities as darkness, reflection, night, rest, contraction, and so on. Neither Yin nor Yang is superior to the other, but, as night turns into day and day into night, each flows into the other in a never-ending cyclical dance. One could not exist without the other.

The concepts of Yin and Yang are often illustrated by a series of tenets. These can best be summarized in the following ways:

  * *Yin and Yang are two phases of one universal cyclical movement.*

All phenomena contain both a Yin aspect and a Yang aspect in continual engagement as part of a larger unity. An example of this is our 24-hour cycle of day and night. As the sun rises and the world changes from Yin to Yang, the quiescent Qi of night slowly transforms into the more active Qi of day. The opposite occurs at sunset when the daylight qualities of Yang slowly give way to the Yin of night.

  * *Any Yin or Yang component can be further subdivided into Yin and Yang components.*

The subdivision of any Yang quality contains elements of both Yang and Yin and the subdivision of any Yin quality contains elements of both Yin and Yang. Using the above example of daybreak, just before the sun breaks over the horizon, the Yin quality of darkness dominates, even though the Yang quality of brightness is slowly increasing. So during a sunrise there exists a slowly changing mixture of Yin and Yang that contains both lightness and darkness. Next, as the sun breaks over the horizon, the Qi of Yang begins to dominate over Yin, and the Qi of Yin slowly recedes as Yang increases.

  * *Yin and Yang mutually create one another.*

The qualities of Yin and Yang cannot be entirely separated. As can be seen in the sunrise example, as Yin diminishes, Yang naturally increases. There is continual interdependence of the varying qualities of Yin and Yang in any natural phenomena. It is the dynamic balance of Qi.

  * *Yin and Yang control one another.*

As the sun rises, the quantity of sunlight that exists at any given time automatically determines, or controls, the amount of darkness present. Within the whole of the day/night cycle, a set quantity of one (darkness or light) naturally predetermines the quantity of the other.

  * *Yin and Yang transform into one another.*

The change of day into night or night into day is a gradual transformation that we experience continually. It is the classic example of the transformation of Yin into Yang and Yang into Yin.

Yin and Yang play a vital role within the context of Chinese medicine by representing the elements of balance one should strive to achieve in maintaining a healthy lifestyle. But this is only one component of the Yin/Yang dynamic. By noting the above tenets, we can see that the Qi of Yin and Yang define all the other aspects of the practice of TCM as well. This includes the signs and symptoms of any disease process, the treatment plan the physician develops, and the modality chosen for treatment. The structures of the body as well are defined into their respective Yin and Yang components.

Table 1 below gives some further examples.

	Yin	Yang
Body	Front	Back
	Interior	Exterior
	Abdomen/Chest	Skin/Muscles
	Below the Waist	Above the Waist
	Structure	Function
Pathology	Chronic Disease	Acute Disease
	Gradual Onset	Rapid Onset
	Coldness	Heat
	Fatigue	Restlessness
	Weak Voice	Loud Voice
Treatment	Long Treatment	Short Treatment
	Herbal Therapy	Acupuncture/Moxa
	More Needles	Fewer Needles
	Dispersion Technique	Tonification Technique

Table 1: Aspects of Yin and Yang

Diagnosis requires careful analysis of Qi as it reflects in the various Yin and Yang components of a disease state. This allows a practitioner to determine the disease pattern correctly and develop a diagnosis and treatment plan. Two traditional yet very different diagnostic models used in this process are the Eight Principles and the Five Element Theory. Both models are complete systems unto themselves yet each also complements the other. The Chinese evolved a worldview that transcended "either/or" thinking and allowed for flexibility and multiple diagnostic frames of reference. They understood that none would be absolutely right for all situations. It is more a matter of determining which is most appropriate for the situation at hand.

THE EIGHT PRINCIPLES

Identifying pathological patterns according to the Eight Principles requires a very precise and thorough grasp of the dynamics of Qi in relation to the cyclical dance of Yin and Yang. The Eight Principles include four pairs of polarities: Interior/Exterior, Cold/Hot, Deficiency/Excess, and, in an overview capacity, Yin/Yang.

Any diseased or imbalanced state of Qi can be categorized according to these Eight Principles and, using this system, a practitioner can unravel complex disease patterns and reduce them to their essential qualities. Let's examine these pairs of principles in greater detail.

Interior/Exterior

This pair indicates the location of the disease or where the major activity of Qi is focused in the body. An interior condition affects the internal organ systems and the bones. With interior conditions the Qi is focused more deeply within the body and usually results from the body's attempt to rebalance internal processes. Exterior conditions mean that the Qi is involved more with the surface areas of the body, such as the skin and muscles. Imbalances of Qi in these areas might manifest as rashes, colds and fevers, shivering, numbness and tingling in the limbs, etc.

Cold/Hot

This pair of the Eight Principles describes the nature of the imbalance. In TCM, Cold is viewed in a couple of ways. The first is simply as a lack of warmth. This often indicates disease states in which the body's Qi is insufficient and not able to keep the body warm. Wrapping in warm clothes helps to alleviate this coldness. The second is that Cold is also viewed as a true entity that can imbed itself in the tissues. This gives rise to a feeling of coldness in which it is difficult to get warm no matter how much one wraps up. Thus Cold patterns usually manifest as slowness, paleness, inability to get warm, shivering, pain, or may even be the cause when an individual appears withdrawn. Hot indicates disease states in which Qi is in a much more active or agitated state. This activity generates heat, generally leading to warm symptoms such as fever, inflammation, red face or eyes, or quick, agitated movements.

Deficiency/Excess

This pair distinguishes between the presence or absence of a pathological factor invading the body, as well as the strength of the body's inherent energies. A deficient condition is characterized by an insufficiency of body Qi or Blood. Many times in deficient conditions a person feels overly tired or cold or, since Qi orchestrates the activity of our different physiological systems, these may not function optimally. On the other hand, an excess condition is characterized by the presence of pathological Qi within the body, such as a cold or flu with accompanying symptoms. It is termed excess because the pathological Qi which has invaded is adding more Qi to the body than is its normal quota.

Yin/Yang

The Yin/Yang pair represents the summation of the other six categories, yet can also describe certain aspects of imbalance that do not fit precisely into the other categories.

THE FIVE ELEMENTS

Another important diagnostic and therapeutic framework in TCM is the Five Elements Theory. This theory evolved from observation of natural phenomena into a system of correspondences that ties all natural processes to five phase relationships. The Five Elements—Wood, Fire, Earth, Metal, and Water—are regarded as energetic qualities inherent in all things. Each element is a symbol that represents a category of related functions or qualities. For example, the Qi of the Wood element is associated with activities of growing or increasing, as wood naturally does in the spring. Fire Qi correlates to activity that has peaked and is ready to decline. Metal Qi represents activities that are decreasing, or declining, and the Qi of Water is associated with activities that have reached a maximum state of decline and are preparing to grow. The Qi of Earth designates centrality or neutrality and is seen as a buffer among the other elements. The Five Elements have symbolic correspondences associated with all aspects of the natural world, as Table 2 on the next page indicates.

A TCM practitioner might use Five Element correspondences to assist in diagnosis. For example, Table 2 shows that the Metal element is associated with the Lungs, nose, skin, autumn, mucus and

	Wood	Fire	Earth	Metal	Water
Yin Organ	Liver	Heart	Spleen	Lungs	Kidney
Yang Organ	Gall Bladder	Sm. Intestines	Stomach	Lg. Intestines	Urinary Bladder
Season	Spring	Summer	Indian Summer	Autumn	Winter
Color	Green	Red	Yellow	White	Black
Odor	Rancid	Scorched	Fragrant	Rotten	Putrid
Direction	East	South	Center	West	North
Climate	Windy	Hot	Damp	Dry	Cold
Emotion	Anger	Joy	Worry	Grief	Fear
Taste	Sour	Bitter	Sweet	Pungent	Salty
Sound	Shout	Laugh	Sing	Weep	Groan
Musical Note	*Chio*	*Chih*	*Kung*	*Shang*	*Yu*
Tissue	Tendons	Blood	Muscles	Skin	Bones
Meat	Chicken	Mutton	Beef	Horse	Pork
Cereal	Wheat	Glutinous Millet	Millet	Rice	Beans
Fluid	Tears	Sweat	Saliva	Mucus	Urine
Sense Organ	Eyes	Tongue	Mouth	Nose	Ears

Table 2: The Five Elements

the color white. Looking at this clinically, we know that in the fall, as the weather cools, people are prone to catching colds. There may be chills or fever (skin), rhinitis (nose/mucus) and often, congestion in the chest (mucus) with cough (Lungs). Many times a pale complexion (color) is also a symptom. These types of correspondences hold true for each phase of the Five Elements, and even though some associations may seem forced, as a whole they are quite useful clinically.

The Qi of each of the Five Elements continually interacts with the others in a variety of sequences. In one of the most commonly used arrangements, the Mutual Production Cycle (see Figure 2), each ele-

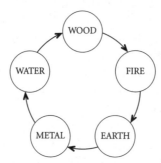

Figure 2: The Mutual Production Cycle

ment moves and blends into the next in the sequential pattern of Wood-Fire-Earth-Metal-Water. This is best exemplified in the patterns of seasonal growth, as depicted below.

Wood, corresponding to spring, turns naturally into Fire, the element of summer. As summer progresses it moves into what we call Indian summer. This corresponds to the element Earth. Indian summer is naturally followed by fall (Metal), and winter (Water) completes the cycle. The cycle begins again when winter changes into spring (Wood). In this scheme each phase smoothly flows into the next and at the same time depends on the previous phase for its own nourishment.

The Mutual Production Cycle is one of many employed within the framework of TCM and is often used to describe clinical processes and relationships that help to formulate appropriate diagnosis and treatment.

Another sequence, the Mutual Control Cycle (see Figure 3), Wood-Earth-Water-Fire-Metal, describes the means by which the different systems of the body harmoniously keep each other in check. A breakdown in this sequence results in one Element overly controlling the

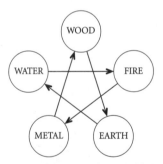

Figure 3: The Mutual Control Cycle

one following it in the sequence. The controlling Element is usually excessive in Qi, or hyperacting. This excessive Qi impinges on the element that it is supposed to control, creating an imbalance. For example, Wood should control Earth to help keep it in balance, but when this relationship is disturbed, for instance by excessive anger (Liver/Wood), a person may become overly pensive or suffer from digestive disorders (Spleen/Earth).

Many acupuncture points correspond to the Five Elements. Using the above example, if Wood (Liver) becomes overactive and dominates the Earth (Spleen), resulting in digestive disorders, the acupuncturist might needle Five Element acupuncture points to calm the Liver Qi and perhaps, if necessary, reinforce the Qi of the Spleen. This treatment would once again bring about a balance between the Wood and Earth elements and alleviate the digestive symptoms.

These two cycles are the most frequently used in TCM. The Five Elements allow us to correlate observed natural phenomena in the macrocosm with the microcosm of human life. In this regard, it can be a very useful tool in understanding people's relationship to the greater whole of the natural world.

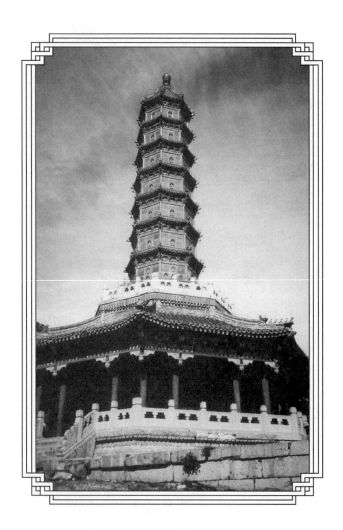

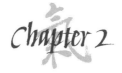

Chapter 2

THEORETICAL FRAMEWORK

When exploring TCM it is important to be able to interpret the metaphorical language. This is one of the more difficult tasks of the TCM practitioner and can take years of experience to perfect. An indepth exploration is beyond the scope of this book; however, a brief description and explanation of some fundamental concepts can enhance our basic understanding. Our exploration will lead to a new way of viewing the functions of the physical body and its relationship to the emotions, the mind and the Spirit.

VITAL SUBSTANCES: QI, BLOOD, SHEN, AND BODY FLUIDS

TCM views physiological processes as the interaction among various vital substances. The quality and quantity of these vital substances, and their ability to smoothly interact and reinforce one another, provide the mechanism for balance within the body. These substances demonstrate varying degrees of materiality, from the most substantial – Blood to the most rarified – Shen, or Spirit. At the foundation of all of the vital substances, however, is the presence of Qi.

Qi

The concept of Qi is perhaps the most difficult of the vital substances to grasp, but also perhaps the most interesting because of its multidimensional nature. We have spoken of its ubiquitousness, of its vital role in the physiological process, maintenance, and development of the human form, and of its more subtle nature in relation to the activity of our mind, emotions, and Spirit. Qi is an enigma, for it is both a noun and a verb, just as light may be described as a particle and a wave. Qi is both the process of unfolding and that which is unfolding. Life is the proliferation of Qi, death its dissolution. Unraveling the mystery of Chinese medicine is the art of understanding the myriad functions and interactions of Qi. Qi is an invisible, fluid force, a dynamic entity weaving diverse and varied patterns through the fabric of our being. The foundation of our health rests on the harmonious integration and balance that Qi provides. Qi dances in our hearts and allows us the full range of our emotions. It stimulates and powers our minds to give us the ability to reason and dream. It integrates the functions of our bodies, which themselves are the material manifestations of this enlivening force. The famous physician Zhang Zai (1020-1077) stated, "If Qi condenses, its visibility becomes effective and physical form appears."

Within the context of TCM, Qi has a number of primary forms and functions that change according to the environment and circumstances that surround it. Qi is the force propelling the blood through the arteries and veins, yet is the very quality of that blood itself. It is the air that enters our lungs as we breathe, yet is the energy the lungs use to inhale and exhale as well as the lung tissue itself. This may appear paradoxical when viewed strictly from the perspective of anatomy and physiology, but when viewed from the perspective of the vital energy that facilitates those physiological processes, it brings new life and depth to them.

Types of Qi

In relation to living organisms, Qi has two primary aspects: 1) the energetic nourishment of the body and the mind, and 2) its indication in the functional activity of all metabolic, emotional, psychological, and spiritual processes. Traditionally a TCM practitioner assesses the various types of Qi when determining our state of health. These have names that define their role within the larger scope of body energetics.

One type of Qi is known as Prenatal Qi. This encompasses the essential qualities of strength, intelligence, constitutional make-up, and vitality that a person inherits from the union of the essences of his or her parents at conception. Aspects of this could be equated to the western concept of DNA. TCM states that Prenatal Qi is stored in the Kidneys and determines our unique individuality, our strengths and weaknesses, gifts and deficits. It is traditionally believed that the amount of Prenatal Qi one inherits is finite, meaning that it cannot be replaced in the course of one's life. The ancients believed that once the vessel holding this precious essence is empty, life ceases. To protect the essence and slow down its depletion, one should strive for balance in one's daily activities. This is the key to longevity as taught through the Chinese classics.

Postnatal Qi is that essential Qi that we obtain from the food we eat and the air we breathe. The higher the quality of the Postnatal Qi we absorb from food and air, the less we draw on our Prenatal Qi to live. Postnatal Qi is extremely important for the quality of our health. The functioning of our digestive system is intricately linked with our ability to extract the refined nutrients from our food. The quality of Postnatal Qi relies not only on the quality of the foods we eat, but also on the optimal functioning of our digestive system, specifically the Spleen and Stomach. The quality of air we breathe and the optimal functioning of the lungs also play an important role.

When Pre and Postnatal Qi combine in the body, they form a more specific type of Qi known as Kidney Essence or Jing. Jing is more fluid and material (Yin), whereas most of the other types of Qi are more energetic and moving (Yang). Jing plays a significant role in physiological functions, especially growth, development, and maturation. It also governs pregnancy and one's ability to conceive.

These three types of Qi determine the foundation of who we are and how we relate to the world. They color our interactions with others and determine how we feel about ourselves. They provide vitality, clarity of thought, emotional stability, and spiritual understanding. However, though foundational, they are not necessarily the workhorses of the Qi realm. Other types of Qi draw from these foundational qualities and have specific responsibilities when it comes to determining our health and outlook on life. Four of the most important and primary of these other types of Qi are Original Qi (*Yuan Qi*), Food Qi (*Gu Qi*), Nutritive Qi (*Ying Qi*) and Defensive Qi (*Wei Qi*).

Original Qi is derived from Kidney Essence. It is the aspect of Qi in the body that provides the catalyst for change. It is a moving force that circulates throughout the entire body and activates all our organ systems. It also facilitates the transformation of one type of Qi into another and helps in the creation of Blood. It is said that we "store" Original Qi in the Kidneys.

Case #1

Jim is an active 48 year old who participates in a number of sports activities as well as maintaining an active social, work and family life. One afternoon while playing basketball he slipped and slightly injured his lower back. This was the most recent of a number of minor injuries to his back that have occurred over the course of his active life.

During the interview Jim told me that after a good night's rest his back would feel much better but then would start to ache as the day progressed. His physician could find no explanation for the back pain because the initial injury that had brought on the problem appeared to have been resolved. Jim was also suffering from some knee pain. This had slowly been developing over the past couple years.

I advised Jim to modify his sports activities during the course of his work with me. We used a combination of acupuncture and other TCM therapies to help resolve his condition. I saw him initially twice a week for three weeks, at which time the pain in his low back had nearly subsided. At this point I changed my treatment approach and saw him only twice a month for another two months.

The lifestyle that Jim was leading, although balanced in many respects, was depleting him of his Kidney Qi. This depletion was being expressed in his lower back and knee pain. The key to this treatment was noticing that Jim felt better when he rested. In other words, when he was not depleting his reservoir of Qi, but allowed it to replenish, he felt better. All the therapies used helped to nourish this underlying deficiency while at the same time strengthen his lower back. Jim also modified his sports activities to put less stress on his back.

It has been three years since the injury that brought Jim to my office. He occasionally still sees me for minor aches and pains, but he is generally healthy and strong. He is still physically active, but has modified his activities to best serve him in promoting his health, not undermine it.

Food Qi is the nutritional essence extracted from the foods we eat. Even more than that, however, food itself is Qi and, as such, has specific energetic properties associated with it such as hot or cold, bitter or sweet, heavy or light, and so on. The nutritional quality and energetic properties of the foods we eat thus determine the quality of our tissues. We literally infuse the energies of what we eat into our being. This is a truth we all intuitively understand, but it is a foundational principle of Chinese medicine. Nutritional therapy is a branch of Chinese herbology and an integral part of TCM. It all boils down to maintaining balance. For example, if you are feeling cold, eat foods that are warming.

Nutritive Qi has the function of general nourishment of the entire body. As such it is closely related to the nourishing quality of blood and flows more in the interior of the body. It is Nutritive Qi that the acupuncturist's needle stimulates when inserted into an acupuncture point.

Defensive Qi protects our body from harmful external factors in our environment. Defensive Qi flows more exteriorly and not only protects us, but helps to nourish, moisten, and warm the skin and muscles. It is in charge of opening and closing our pores and regulates sweating, which in turn, helps us maintain our body temperature. Defensive Qi is rather like wearing a protective coat over our physical form as a defensive force field.

As we have seen in these examples, various types of Qi attend to specific physiological functions. However, when we look beyond these examples and examine the numerous activities of bodily Qi when taken as a whole, they can be broken down and summarized into the following six energetic categories:

1. **Catalyzing:** Qi transforms itself into other forms

2. **Transporting:** Qi moves itself and blood throughout the body/mind/spirit

3. **Stabilizing:** Qi holds organs in their place and keeps blood within the vessels

4. **Raising:** Qi rises upward in the body to nourish the mind and spirit

5. **Protecting:** Qi defends the body from external pathogenic factors

6. **Warming:** Qi warms the body, both internally and on the surface

The concept of Qi is difficult to translate, but by contemplating these functions and the energetics of Qi, the scope and mystery may be more deeply appreciated.

Blood

Blood is not only the red fluid that flows through our arteries and veins but is also a condensed form of Qi, one that is very material in nature. Chinese medicine teaches that, "Qi is the commander of Blood and Blood is the mother of Qi." This denotes the interdependency and complementarity of Qi and Blood. In this statement Qi is considered the Yang component of the Blood, giving it movement and vitality, whereas the fluid itself is considered the substantive, nourishing Yin component. As is often the case with TCM, it can be difficult to see where one function or quality leaves off and another begins. Qi and Blood. Are they the same? Yes. Are they different? Yes. But one thing can be stated for sure, Qi and Blood are intimately bound and rely on each other for their very existence. In a living being, they are inseparable.

Case #2

Amy was a professional dancer. Nine months before she came to see me she had been involved in a minor traffic accident that had left her with upper back and neck pain, especially on her right side. She had tried conventional therapies, including chiropractic, but the pain and stiffness, although improved, still persisted.

Diagnostic evaluation revealed that Amy had severe areas of tension and sore spots between her spine and the right scapula on her back. When these areas were palpated, the pain radiated up into her neck and across the back of her right shoulder.

I determined that she was suffering from Stagnation of Qi and Blood in specific meridians that flowed through her neck and back area. These blockages in the meridians were causing the pain and stiffness. I selected a series of acupuncture points that would help to remove the blockages in the affected meridians. Most points were in the local area of pain, but some were at distal locations away from the site of injury. The distal sites were near her ankles, knees, and the side of her right hand. I also applied warmth to the injured area. This technique also helps move stagnant Qi. The needles were left in for about twenty-five minutes. After removing the needles I used a specific acupressure technique that also helps to remove blockages and helps nourish the locally injured area by increasing blood flow to it. I saw Amy eight times over the course of four weeks, varying each treatment as the condition changed and slowly resolved. By the end of the eighth session she was pain free and enjoying dancing again. A follow-up phone call two months later revealed that she was having no more trouble with her upper back and neck.

Shen

Shen, best translated as Spirit, Mind, or Consciousness, is the most rarefied form of Qi that embodies us. It is that spiritual component of who we are and is reflected in our eyes. It is our halo, our aura. The TCM practitioner examines the Shen of an individual by noting the brightness of the eyes, the clarity of speech and thought, and the luminescence around the body. Shen is traditionally said to reside in the Heart. Since the Heart also circulates Qi and Blood throughout the body to nourish every cell, we might expand this concept to support the idea that the subtle consciousness of Spirit is also transported to every cell. Thus Spirit, or consciousness, permeates every tissue of our bodies.

Body Fluids

Body Fluids, other than Blood, also moisten and nourish the body. Chinese medicine depicts two types of Body Fluids. The relatively clear and watery type is said to circulate in the exterior of the body, nourishing and moistening the skin and muscles. The more turbid and heavy type circulates much deeper. It moistens and nourishes the joints, spine, and brain, as well as the sense organs - eyes, nose, ears, and mouth. The Body Fluids are produced from the activity of the Spleen and Stomach absorbing and dispersing the nutrients from what we eat and drink.

ORGAN SYSTEMS

The internal organ systems of TCM are viewed in quite a different manner than they are in western medicine. TCM attributes energetic qualities to each of the major organs or organ systems. Not only does an organ provide a specific physiological activity with complex functional relationships, but each has a unique spirit that transcends physiology. Each organ is aligned with a specific emotion or state of consciousness. This energetic perspective thus weaves our consciousness and state of mental health directly into our physical form. The TCM practitioner knows that if any one of our emotions is out of balance for too long, it eventually presents as a disease state in the respective organ system. Conversely, an organ system that is persistently unbalanced eventually expresses itself through the mental or emotional states.

Chinese medicine categorizes the internal organs as either Yin or Yang. Yin organs (Zang) are considered solid and store the various Vital Substances. They are primarily responsible for producing, maintaining, transforming, and moving the Vital Substances and are the energetic core of the internal organ systems. The functional and spiritual qualities of the Yin organs take precedence over the Yang organs. The Yang organs (Fu) are hollow and are responsible for receiving, digesting, transporting, and excreting. The Yin/Yang balance of the organ systems is maintained by pairing a Yin organ with a Yang organ. These Zang-Fu pairings, although not always physiologically complementary, are energetically related.

Below is a partial list of the energetic natures and correspondences followed by a list of common imbalances for each of the major Yin organ systems.

Lungs: Metal element, coupled with Large Intestine (Yang)

The Lungs are said to govern Qi and respiration by extracting Qi from the air we breathe and exhaling "dirty" Qi (carbon dioxide). The Lungs are associated with the skin and body hair and are also in control of dispersing and descending Qi. This means that the Lungs move Qi downward in the body and at the same time disperse Qi to the surface of the skin to help protect us (Defensive Qi). The nose is the opening for the Lungs and is associated with our sense of smell. The Lungs are said to house the corporeal soul. The emotion associated with the Lungs is grief.

Imbalances are usually Lung problems, such as shortness of breath, sinusitis, allergies, cough, asthma, dry skin and spontaneous sweating. The Lungs are the most external of the Yin organs and are therefore more subject to external influences, such as cold, wind, heat, dryness.

Spleen: Earth element, coupled with Stomach (Yang)

The Spleen is said to transform and transport Qi from the nutrients that we eat. Because of this function, the Spleen is considered the foundation of digestion. The energy of the Spleen ascends, meaning that it moves Qi upward in the body. This helps to hold Blood in the vessels and organs in their place. In TCM a prolapsed organ indicates a deficiency of Spleen Qi. The Spleen also controls the strength of the muscles and the four limbs. The mouth is the opening for the Spleen and is the means by which we taste the foods we eat. The Spleen is also said to govern our intellect. The mental state associated with the Spleen is pensiveness and worry.

Imbalances include digestive disorders such as obesity, food cravings, nausea, loose stools, abdominal fullness and organ prolapse. Other imbalances may present as excessive thinking, either as overwork or worry, and fatigue.

Case #3

Sharon, 26, had a severe case of insomnia that seemed to be getting worse with each passing month. She also suffered from occasional loose stools, PMS, and had recently been diagnosed by her physician as being anemic. Most of these conditions had been with her for at least three years. She was a full-time student and worked part-time as a waitress to help meet expenses. She had erratic eating habits.

When I first met Sharon her demeanor was calm and she appeared both tired and frail. The diagnostic interview revealed a lack of Qi in her digestive functions resulting in an inability to absorb and utilize the Qi from the foods she ate. This corresponded to the western diagnosis of anemia. She also mentioned that when she was younger she had had severe menstrual bleeding but now was having very short periods with little bleeding. Assessment of all these factors led me to a traditional Chinese diagnosis of deficiency of Blood in her system. This condition was leading to her insomnia and lethargy and was a direct result of her inability to absorb the Qi in her food.

In treating Sharon it was important to strengthen her digestive system which, in turn, would strengthen the vitality of her Blood. Treat-

ment modalities were acupuncture, heat (moxibustion) and herbal therapy. I advised her to regulate her eating habits, and generally, to eat warming foods such as hot soups and hot teas, while curtailing her intake of cold drinks, raw foods, and ice cream. Consistent ingestion of raw and cold foods stress the body's digestive capabilities. Warm foods aid in digestion.

This treatment strategy resolved her loose stools within a few weeks, and although her insomnia improved during this time, it was not until about two months after treatment that she started to notice a real change in her sleeping pattern. Treatment also focused indirectly on her PMS symptoms and her anemia. It was another two months before her periods became more normal and her anemia was no longer of medical concern.

In this case, strengthening her digestion allowed her body to take in the required energy needed to produce more Blood. The lack of Blood failed to nourish the mind and brought on the insomnia.

Kidneys: Water element, coupled with Urinary Bladder (Yang)

The Kidneys store Prenatal Qi and Jing, and control birth, growth, maturation, and sexuality. The Kidneys are considered the foundation of life. In TCM the Kidneys govern the bones, bone marrow, the brain, the back, and the spinal cord. In concert with the Lungs, the Kidneys control the reception of Qi and together they facilitate breathing. The ears are considered the openings for the Kidneys, and Kidney energy effects our ability to hear. The Kidneys are also associated with the hair on the head. The Kidneys are said to govern the will and passion for life and maintain life's "pilot light" (Prenatal Qi), which dissipates with age. The emotion associated with the Kidneys is fear.

Imbalances include retarded development, back pain, sore knees, deafness and tinnitus, urinary problems, prostatitis, reduced sexual drive, fatigue, night sweating, dizziness, and poor memory or concentration.

Heart: Fire element, coupled with Small Intestine (Yang)

The Heart is said to govern Blood and circulation. According to TCM, the transformation of Qi into Blood takes place in the Heart, as well as in the bones. The Heart manifests in the complexion and is associated with the tongue. The Heart also stores the Shen—the Spirit or Mind. Because of the intimate connection with the Mind, the Heart is strongly associated with consciousness and is said to be the sovereign ruler of the body. The emotion associated with the Heart is joy. Imbalances include heart disease, insomnia, dream-disturbed sleep, anxiety, palpitations, mania, and other mental disturbances.

Liver: Wood element, coupled with Gall Bladder (Yang)

The Liver stores Blood when one is resting and releases it for activity where it is needed, as when exercising. It also regulates Blood volume and is intimately associated with menstruation. One of the main functions of the Liver is to ensure the smooth flow of Qi throughout the body. This function has a strong emotional component, depicted by the TCM phrase "Stagnant Liver Qi," which is the hallmark of mood swings and irritability. The Liver also controls the tendons and is reflected in the fingernails by their color and strength. The eyes are considered the openings for the Liver and are associated with our ability to see. The Liver is also said to govern the psychospiritual nature and ethereal soul. The emotion associated with the Liver is anger.

Imbalances include depression, anger, frustration, headaches, tendinitis, hypertension, eye problems, heartburn, PMS, fibroids, muscular tension, tics, tremors, spasms, or moving pains.

Case #4

Mary was experiencing a lot of stress in her life. The recent addition of headaches to her already difficult working situation did not help matters. Mary was angry that she had recently been passed over for a promotion and felt frustrated at not being able to communicate with her boss. The headaches started soon after her feelings of frustration.

Mary's signs and symptoms – frustration, unexpressed anger, insomnia, dizziness, headaches, and emotional fatigue – indicated that her emotional state was at the root of her headache problem.

I treated Mary by treating her anger. The energy of anger was rising in her and causing excess amounts of Qi to gather in her head. This resulted in the headaches, insomnia, and dizziness. I chose points that calmed her spirit and smoothed her emotions. I suggested she develop avenues of communication with her boss and perhaps take an anger management course.

I saw Mary twice a week for two weeks, during which time the headaches slowly subsided. A follow-up call three weeks later revealed that Mary had indeed enrolled in an anger management course and was also in the process of interviewing for another job.

Pericardium: Fire element, coupled with Triple Burner* (Yang)

The Pericardium protects the Heart from external pathogenic influences. It is said to influence a person's relations with other people. Many functions of the Pericardium mirror those of the Heart, including its emotional associations.

The Yang organ systems, because of their subordinate stature, are not generally given specific energetic functions, but share the functions of their respective Yin organs. All organ relationships have both psychological and physiological aspects. Some relationships are more psychological, as that between the Heart and Small Intestine. Others resonate more with physiological processes, for example that between the Spleen and Stomach, both of which are involved with digestion.

MERIDIAN AND POINT THEORY

Meridians

The Chinese consider all parts of the universe to be interrelated and often refer to the body as if it were a landscape. The rivers of the earth, which allow for communication between its various regions, are reflected in the body, the microcosm again reflecting the macrocosm. From this thinking, and through centuries of empirical observation, the meridian and point system of Chinese medicine was developed. Figures 4 through 6 represent the flows of the meridians as they traverse the surface of the body.

Many acupuncture texts depict the meridians as lines drawn on the body, much as a river is drawn on a map. In many respects this representation is valid for it shows where the river, or meridian, flows and, in the case of acupuncture, which acupuncture points are located along its course. But the meridian system is much more com-

---

*Also called triple warmer, triple energizer, or San Jiao, is one of the 12 primary meridians and corresponds to the upper, middle and lower portions of the body.

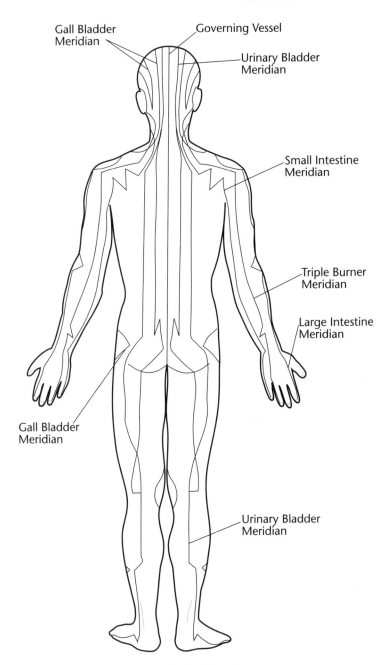

Figure 4: Back Meridian System

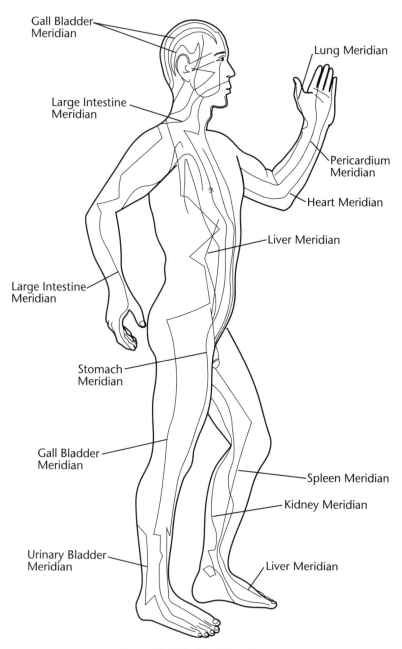

Gall Bladder Meridian

Lung Meridian

Large Intestine Meridian

Pericardium Meridian

Heart Meridian

Liver Meridian

Large Intestine Meridian

Stomach Meridian

Gall Bladder Meridian

Spleen Meridian

Kidney Meridian

Urinary Bladder Meridian

Liver Meridian

Figure 5: Side Meridian System

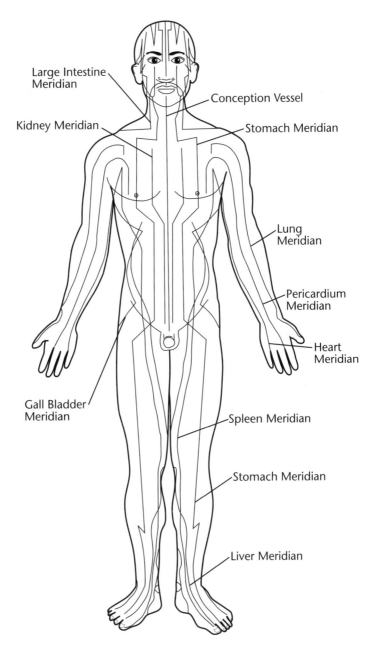

Figure 6: Front Meridian System

plex and poetic than this representative line on the body, just like the line on the map does not do justice to a river. Within a river are currents, eddies, smooth rocks, and aquatic life forms. The water within the river does not stop at the river's bank, but permeates the land deeply along its entire course. Sometimes the river is shallow, sometimes it runs deep. These images also hold true for the fluidity of Qi running through a meridian. Depending on the muscles and tissues it traverses, a meridian might also run deep or shallow. In some areas it might spread over the surface of the skin and in other places become more narrow. At one point it might run quickly, at another more slowly. A meridian has an energetic signature that reflects the portion of the body it traverses, its associated organ system, and the quality of the Qi that flows along its course. The meridians, as conduits of Qi, permeate the entire body. The best known are the twelve primary meridians that run near the surface of the body. They are arranged symmetrically on each side of the body, the left side directly mirroring the right. These primary meridians also have branches that penetrate deeply into the interior of the body to connect with their respective Yin/Yang organ systems. Each meridian is named after the internal organ it is associated with, for example, the Lung meridian, the Large Intestine Meridian, the Liver Meridian, and so on. Thus we can see that a meridian is not separate from the organ, but is an extension of that organ system's energetics. When an organ system's Qi becomes imbalanced, that energetic disharmony is echoed by the respective meridian and eventually is reflected on the surface of the body in the region the meridian traverses. Conversely, an imbalance in a meridian can be mirrored in its respective organ system.

There are many types of meridians. In addition to the twelve primary meridians associated with each of the twelve organ systems, two additional meridians traverse the midline of the front (Ren/Conception Vessel) and the back (Du/Governing Vessel) of the body. It is on these fourteen meridians that the major acupuncture points are located. There also exists groupings of other channels that connect to or branch from the primary meridians. Each of these subsets have specific functions that augment the activities of the fourteen primary meridians. Some of these are minor channels that distribute Qi from the primary channels to finer and finer regions of the body. Eventually, every cell is vitalized by the Qi within the meridian system. This complex system of subdivision is much like the blood circulatory system which proceeds from major arteries down to the smallest capillaries.

Acupuncture Points

The acupuncture points, or xue (pronounced shway), meaning "hole," are minute locations on the skin where the Qi flowing in the meridians emerges. Using the analogy of the river, the acupuncture points can be viewed as whirlpools. These whirlpools allow for communication between the surface of the body and the deeper currents of Qi. It is through the application of acupuncture needles at the acupuncture points that the Qi within the meridians is influenced. This in turn affects the local musculoskeletal area or deeper internal organs associated with that meridian. The systems of meridians and points is a vast communications network that unifies and integrates the workings of the entire body.

Each acupuncture point has a variety of functions and, depending on how it is needled, these different functions may be modified. For example, a point may regulate Qi but, depending upon the needling technique applied, the Qi flow may be reinforced in the meridian or it may be dispersed. Many acupuncture point names refer to the points location or reflect its energetic nature. *Xiyan*, for example,

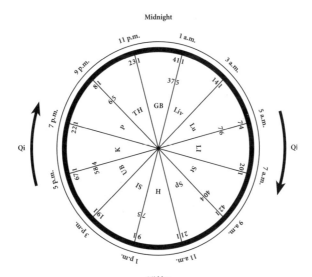

Figure 7: 24 Hour Cycle

means " Eyes of the Knee," and is located in the hollow on either side of the kneecap. *Qihai*, "Sea of Qi," denotes a point slightly below the navel that functions as a reservoir of Qi. The body reflects a diverse landscape where the acupuncture points are the signposts along the rivers of Qi.

The 24-Hour Cycle of Rhythms

The Qi that flows through the meridian system and nourishes the internal organs does so in an organized manner. Each of the twelve meridians and respective organs has a maximum energy flow of two hours within a twenty-four hour cycle. Each is associated with a specific time of day. For example, the cycle begins at 3:00 a.m. when the Qi begins to flow through the Lung Meridian, peaking at 4:00 a.m., then ebbing until 5:00 a.m. Then Qi moves into the Large Intestine Meridian. This flow continues until the Qi has moved through all twelve organ systems and their meridians (see Figure 7). This does not mean that the other systems are lacking Qi when one is at its maximum. It simply means that each organ system and its meridian get a maximal boost of Qi every twenty-four hours.

The Causes of Disharmony

An imbalance within the energetic systems of the body, either in the organs or the meridians, eventually gives rise to illness. Many factors, both from within the body and from external sources, can destabilize and weaken the Qi and Blood.

We know that when an individual has strong, balanced Qi and Blood, disease has more difficulty gaining a foothold. Conversely, deficient or stagnant Qi or Blood disturbs the balance of Yin and Yang of the body and creates a weakened condition from which disease or pain is more likely to occur. Internal causes of disease vary and include injury or trauma, poor diet or malabsorption of food, congenital disorders, emotional imbalances, overexertion, or excessive sexual activity. These conditions, if chronic or severe enough, can greatly impact the body's ability to use Qi optimally, thus impairing the functions of the organ systems.

Chinese medicine also attributes the Qi of climatic factors as causes of disharmony and illness. Traditionally these are the Six External Pathogenic Influences, or "Six Evils:" Wind, Cold, Dampness, Dryness, Heat and Summer-Heat. The Qi of the environment is seen to be pathologic only if it invades the body. For instance, a specific climatic factor may invade the surface tissues of the body where the meridians lie. If it penetrates the meridian system it may then travel deeper into the body to disrupt the Qi of the muscles or the organ systems. Once in the body this pathogenic Qi mimics the corresponding atmospheric element in nature. This results in specific clinical signs and symptoms for each of the Six Evils. Onset of symptoms is usually quite sudden, but they can also become chronic if unattended to.

Wind

Wind is an atmospheric condition that is Yang in nature. In the body it is associated with the Liver and is often the vehicle through which the other climatic factors invade the body. For example, you may hear your practitioner referring to Wind-Cold or Wind-Heat. These are instances where either Cold or Heat has entered the body along with Wind resulting in a cold or flu. Just as atmospheric wind moves one branch of a tree and then another, internal Wind creates conditions in which signs or symptoms move from one area of the body to another. Wind also brings rapid onset of disorders. Symptoms may change rapidly when Wind is involved. Wind is also associated with itching, twitches, tremors, and convulsions. Paradoxically, Wind can also cause paralysis.

Case #5

Carlos had been suffering from a cold for nearly a week when he first came to see me. He had been out fishing one early, gusty morning and came down with a cold the next day. His signs and symptoms included chills, headache, a scratchy throat, runny nose, and general body aches.

My diagnosis was Wind-Cold invasion and I treated him by expelling the Wind-Cold trapped in the surface of his body and also by reinforcing his Lung Qi.

Treatment consisted of needling acupuncture points on his hands, wrists, and the back of his neck. I gave Carlos an herbal tea that helped him to sweat and expel the Wind-Cold through his pores. The treatment was successful and he was back to normal in two days. I also advised Carlos to keep himself wrapped up warmly, especially around his neck, while fishing in the cooler early mornings.

Cold

Cold is Yin in nature, associated with the Kidneys, and can injure the Yang Qi of the body. Cold enters the meridians and channels, impedes the flow of Qi, and causes chilliness, stiffness, and pain. It is most often associated with Wind-Cold conditions and manifests as the common cold or flu. Cold has a strong affinity for muscles and joints and some types of arthritis are referred to as Cold Stagnation Arthritis. Cold can also occur deep within the body due to a lack of Yang, or warmth. This type of Cold can be brought on by exposure to cold, eating too much raw and cold foods, over-exertion or excessive sexual activity. These latter two deplete the body of Yang Qi, or in this case, warmth.

Case #6

John was a very healthy older gentleman with a passion for playing golf in the early morning. During his recent games he started noticing an annoying pain on the inside of his left elbow. He came to see me in the late fall after he'd had this condition for about two months and it started affecting his game.

Palpation revealed a very sore spot on the inside of his left elbow. I chose acupuncture for the main therapy along with rice grain moxibustion. I chose acupuncture points near the site of pain as well as distal points on the forearm and hand along meridians that crossed over the area of pain and another down by his knee. I applied rice grain moxibustion at the most painful site on the inside of the elbow.

John responded well to treatment and saw me only four times over the course of two weeks. I recommended to him that he curtail his golfing for at least the two weeks we were working together.

My diagnosis for this condition was obstruction of Qi due to overuse and Cold invasion in the meridians. The acupuncture points chosen helped to move the obstruction in the channels. This was partially caused by Cold lodged in the meridians at the site of the elbow. The use of the rice grain moxibustion helped not only to move the energy along the meridians, but also to resolve the Cold as well. I suggested to John that he keep his arms warm at all times when he was out golfing in the colder weather.

A follow-up phone call three weeks later revealed that his "golfers elbow" had been resolved. He was also playing less due to inclement

*weather and was looking forward to the spring. I am sure this re-
prieve from constant use of his elbow also aided in the healing.*

Dampness

Dampness, associated with the Spleen, is the most difficult pathogenic factor to treat. Dampness is Yin in nature and thus tends to
injure the Yang Qi of the body. As an external pathogenic factor,
Dampness occurs when an individual spends too much time in a damp
environment or eats too much sweet or rich food. Being caught in
the rain, living in damp quarters, wearing wet clothes or chronically
working under damp conditions can also foster Dampness in the body.
The clinical manifestations vary depending upon their location. Generally, Dampness is heavy and tends to move downward. Conditions
such as diarrhea, edema, obesity, phlegm accumulation, and vaginal
discharge are attributed to Dampness.

Dryness

Dryness is Yang in nature, associated with the Lungs, and tends to
injure Yin Qi. This pathogenic factor is created by very dry environmental conditions. These can either be outside, as in the desert, or in
a building in which central heating or cooling cause a very dry environment. Dryness generally presents clinically as dry throat and
mouth, dry cough, dry lips and skin, and dry stools or constipation.

Heat

Heat, sometimes referred to as Fire and associated with the Heart,
is a very active Yang element that can easily injure the Yin Qi of the
body. Heat naturally presents as signs and symptoms of heat within
the body, such as fever, inflammations, red eyes, flushing, and sensations of warmth. Clinically, Heat can also manifest as red skin erup-
tions, yellow mucus, hemorrhaging, and sore throat.

Summer Heat

Summer Heat is also Yang in nature but is less severe than Heat. It
also injures the Yin Qi. Summer Heat is an external climatic influence that always results from exposure to extreme heat. Its signs and
symptoms include sudden high fever with heavy sweating and diarrhea. Summer Heat often depletes the Body Fluids and causes dryness.

Pathogenic factors often occur in combination, whether internally induced over time due to deficiency or stagnation, or externally induced by environmental factors, for example, Wind-Heat, Deficient Blood that gives rise to Heat, anger creating Liver-Wind, and so on. The patterns of disharmony these combinations create have a variety of clinical presentations.

DIAGNOSTIC METHODS:
LOOKING, LISTENING/SMELLING, ASKING AND TOUCHING

The practitioner of TCM uses many of the same diagnostic methods that traditional western medicine uses. Many of the approaches, however, differ greatly, most notably observation of the tongue and pulse taking. Like western physicians, TCM practitioners must be receptive and have keenly developed diagnostic skills in order to discern the subtle nuances of disharmony that the client presents. TCM looks beyond isolated signs and symptoms by viewing the individual as a dynamically integrated whole. Presenting signs and symptoms weave together into patterns or syndromes that create an energetic profile of the patient. Patience is another potent quality a skilled TCM practitioner exhibits. A still and receptive mind fosters the intuitive process that allows for a deeply empathetic understanding of the patient's Qi.

Traditionally there are Four Methods, or Examinations, that the practitioner uses to gather information for diagnosis and treatment. These Four Examinations are Looking, Listening/Smelling, Asking, and Touching. Each method has many levels of application and uses a different sense for gathering information and interpreting the Qi of the patient.

Looking

In Chinese medical history there is a story of a famous physician who was renowned throughout China for his skills in the art of observation. As a result, many students sought him out as a teacher.

Arriving at the gates of the physician's school, a student was greeted by a servant, offered tea, and told that the teacher would be with him shortly. However, while waiting, the student was presented with a dead fish and asked to write down his observations of it. This was not a pleasant task, and many students felt insulted and left. Others complied and diligently wrote down their observations. However, when after many hours the teacher failed to appear, many of them also left. A few determined students remained, continuing to observe the fish. They may have noticed the slight variations in the size and shape of the scales and how differently they overlapped depending on their position on the body. And they may have noticed the dozens of delicate colors reflected in those scales or the way the tail became transparent as it tapered to its end. Perhaps they began to see the subtle changes as the fish started slowly to decompose. Days passed, perhaps weeks, and the students continued their meticulous observation of the fish as it slowly changed. It was only when a student completed the task of patiently documenting the decomposition of the fish that he was allowed to study further with the teacher. These students became the most highly respected physicians in China because of their impeccable ability to see that which is not normally seen by the untrained eye.

The skill of observation includes noting the general appearance and vitality of an individual. General appearance includes such things as demeanor, posture, facial expression, muscle tone, and the quality of spirit, or Shen, presented by the individual. The practitioner takes note of all observable aspects of the person from their fingernails to the texture and coloring of their skin.

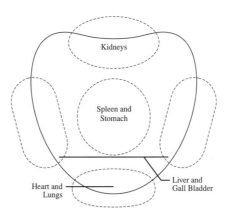

Figure 8: Tongue Diagnosis

Observing the tongue is a very important part of Chinese diagnosis. It reflects the condition of Qi and Blood in the internal organs of the body (see Figure 8). The tongue shape, color, coating, moisture, and texture are all taken into account during diagnosis. Figure 8 depicts the locations on the tongue that are associated with various organ systems. Any variation in normal tongue appearance at any of these specific areas may indicate an imbalance in that particular organ system. The tongue is also observed as a whole. For example, if a patient presents with a tongue that is particularly pale, it may lead to the TCM diagnosis of Deficient Blood. If the tongue coating, or fur, is thick and yellow it may indicate excess heat in the body. A tongue that is extra moist and has a white coating may indicate Cold in the body; cracks on the tongue may indicate the presence of heat; and so on.

Listening/Smelling

The Chinese written language does not differentiate between listening and smelling, thus these two terms are represented by the same pictograph in Chinese. This method of diagnosis focuses the practitioner's attention on the quality of Qi in the person's voice as well as the quality of Qi in their breathing. Qualities of coughing are also noted, as well as any unusual odors that may be present. The practitioner listens for any hints that can give more information as to the underlying cause of a disharmony. For example, an individual with a weak voice may be diagnosed with a condition of Deficient Lung Qi. A person with a loud cough might be diagnosed as having an Excess condition, whereas someone with a weak cough might have a Deficient condition.

Asking

The third Examination, Asking, is one of the most important sources of gathering information. Here the practitioner asks questions, as would a Western physician, about the patient's past medical history, present condition, general lifestyle, and emotional state. Traditionally there are ten areas of inquiry, including asking about sensations of Hot or Cold, perspiration, urine/stool, diet and appetite, sleep, areas and quality of pain, headaches, and dizziness. Asking the patient about their general energy level is also important because it helps the practitioner determine how much Qi the patient has available to aid in their healing process.

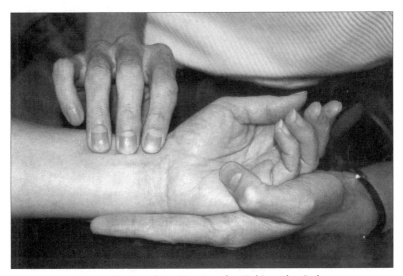

Figure 9: Hand Positioning for Taking the Pulse

Touching

The last of the Four Examinations is Touching. It too is an extremely important process for gathering information. Palpating different areas of the body can give the practitioner information about imbalances both superficially and deep within the body. Many times specific points or meridian sections are tender to the touch due to a disharmony of Qi from deep within the body. The quality of tenderness – for example, dull, sharp, radiating, and so on – will help to determine the appropriate type of therapy.

	Superficial Pulse	**Deep Pulse**
Left Wrist	Small Intestine Gall Bladder Urinary Bladder	Heart Liver Kidney Yin
Right Wrist	Large Intestine Stomach Triple Burner	Lung Spleen Kidney Yang

Table 3: Pulse Positions and Organ Associations

One area of palpatory diagnosis, feeling the radial pulse on the thumb side of each wrist, is of special interest to practitioners of TCM. Pulse diagnosis gives detailed information on the state of the health and Qi of the internal organs as well as the energetic status of the entire body. Pulse diagnosis is extremely subtle and complex. The pulse is felt at superficial and deep levels at three locations on each wrist (see Figure 9 and Table 3). When palpating the pulse, the practitioner focuses on its rate, depth, strength, quality, rhythm, and length. Traditionally, there are twenty-seven pulse types, each one having specific indications that relate to a Qi disharmony in the body. For example, a person whose pulse feels slower than normal may have a cold condition affecting their body, whereas a faster pulse may indicate heat. A pulse that is felt only very deeply usually indicates that the Qi of the body is focused internally, whereas someone whose pulse is felt only very near the surface of the skin may be activating their Protective Qi in order to fight off a cold or flu. Pulses can be big or thin, soft or tight; they may feel fluid or taut or be regular or irregular in their rhythm. Each pulse quality can be combined with others to create a complex system of correspondences and a variety of diagnostic possibilities. For example, a pulse can be slow, deep, and taut. This presentation might indicate a cold and painful condition deep in the body. Or a patient might present with a pulse that is thin and rapid. This might lead to the diagnosis of Deficient Blood with accompanying Heat.

Through focused attention and practice, the practitioner can learn to read the subtleties of Qi dynamics and may even perceive imbalances before they appear as physical complaints.

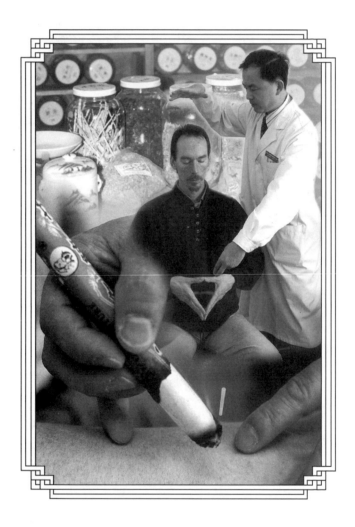

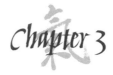

Chapter 3

MODALITIES FOR TREATMENT

Over the centuries, TCM practitioners have developed therapeutic strategies for stimulating and rebalancing the Qi of the body. Today in China these therapies are divided into four main categories: acupuncture, body work, herbology, and medical Qi Gong. During treatment, a TCM practitioner may draw on all of these modalities in combination or may use only one of them at a time. The choice is determined by the condition being treated and the modality that will have the most therapeutic effect. This chaper covers the main therapeutic modalities of TCM and gives the reader an understanding of how and why they are used.

MEDICINE IN CHINA TODAY

Today in most Chinese hospitals, acupuncture, herbology, medical Qi-Gong and tuina (body work) all have their own departments and the doctors employed in these departments work side by side with doctors in the western medical departments. It is an environment of mutual cooperation, trust, and respect. Such a climate of cooperation has created a health care delivery system that incorporates many aspects of a wholistic system. It is a wise blending of western technologies and eastern energetics. The patient is the ultimate recipient of this cooperative effort.

The Chinese people hold the view that activities that enhance health and thus prevent illness are a key to maintaining good health. These healthful activities, or regimens, include proper diet and nutritional knowledge based on Chinese herbs, movement therapies such as Taiji and Qi Gong, meditation, and acupuncture/acupressure for immune enhancement. As we have seen, Oriental medical philosophy is based on maintaining a healthy balance of Yin Qi and Yang Qi in relationship to the earth, community, family, and one's own self nurturing. By cultivating a healthy lifestyle through specific daily activities, the Oriental people have given us many guiding principles for our understanding and employment of preventative medicine.

ACUPUNCTURE

In the West, acupuncture, with its accompanying techniques of moxibustion and cupping, (see Figures 14 and 17) is the most popular of the therapies of TCM. Acupuncture is used primarily when a patient falls ill, experiences pain, or feels out of balance. It is also used as a preventative medicine because it strengthens the body's immune system. During an acupuncture treatment, fine stainless steel needles are inserted into the skin at very specific points. The acupuncture needles are sterile and are disposed of after each treatment.

The needling techniques used in acupuncture are analogous to the mechanisms used in some irrigation systems. At certain points

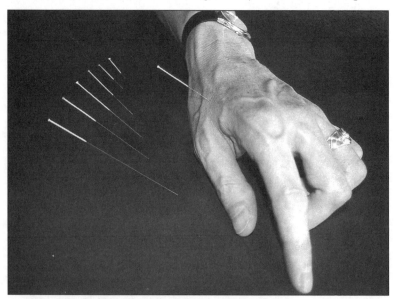

Figure 10: Variety of Acupuncture Needles

an excess of water flow may be drained from a canal into a field where water is needed. Likewise, water may be diverted into a canal from a field that is already flooded. The flow of Qi in the meridians is very similar to this canal or river analogy. The inserted acupuncture needle contacts and stimulates the Qi flowing in the meridians and either increases or diminishes its strength, whichever is appropriate for the treatment.

Most patients feel little sensation on needle insertion due to the fineness of the needle's point. Whereas a standard hollow hypodermic needle used for injections cuts the skin when inserted, acupuncture needles simply separate the tissues with their sharp conical points. After insertion the patient may feel sensations of heaviness, dullness, tingling, or warmth. This is an indication that the Qi in the meridian has been tapped. These sensations may be localized at the insertion site or may be felt traveling along the course of the acupuncture meridian. This sensation is traditionally called obtaining Qi or "deQi" and is an important part of the therapeutic action of acupuncture. This sensation is the movement of the Qi within the body and indicates the potential effectiveness of the treatment.

Choosing the correct acupuncture points is another important key in acupuncture therapy. Each acupuncture point has characteristic functions that, when stimulated, influence the Qi in the meridians in specific ways. The combination of points chosen and the way those points are stimulated is a major factor in how effective an acupuncture treatment is. Some treatments require only two or three points, whereas other treatments may require using a dozen or more acupuncture points. The number of points chosen may also vary from treatment to treatment. The Chinese have an old adage, "You never treat the same patient twice." This means that we mirror nature and the seasons and that our Qi is constantly moving and in flux. Our physiology, as well as our emotional state and mental processes, are different with each passing moment. This is why the practitioner of Chinese medicine may vary the treatment each time, for in each treatment we are treating an energetically different individual.

Acupuncture needles may be left in the skin for 20 or 30 minutes or may be removed immediately after the sensation of Qi is felt. The technique used is determined by the effect that the acupuncturist is trying to achieve. Most practitioners have the patient lying down during a treatment, although accessing different acupuncture points may require the patient to be sitting.

Acupuncture needles vary in length and width (see Figure 10). The most commonly used needles are only about 1" to 1 1/2" in length. The depth of needle insertion usually depends on the site being needled. Some areas are more fleshy, such as the buttocks, legs, and upper arms, and would naturally require deeper needle insertion because the meridians run deeper at these locations. Other areas, such as the face, hands, and feet, which have much less tissue, call for a more shallow needling technique.

Intradermal needles are only a fraction of an inch in length and are often taped onto the skin after they are inserted. They can be worn for a number of days. They cause no discomfort and provide constant stimulation to the acupuncture point over the time that they are worn.

Acupuncture therapists often use microacupuncture systems, for example, the systems on the ear, the face, the hand, the foot, the scalp, and the orbit surrounding the eye. A microacupuncture system is one in which the entire body is represented over a small portion of the skin, such as the ear (see Figure 11).

Acupuncture is applied to the specific site within the microsystem that corresponds to the region of the body that is out of balance. In

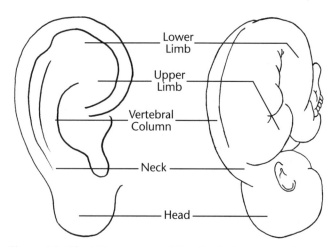

Figure 11: The Microsystem of the Ear is Represented as an Inverted Fetus

this way the entire body can be treated using just the microacupuncture system. In the United States, ear (auricular) acupuncture is the most widely used microsystem because it has shown remarkable results in treating drug and alcohol addiction through inhibiting cravings and aiding the body in detoxification.

ACUPRESSURE

Many styles of acupressure have evolved throughout Asia, but in China the most common is tuina (twee´-nah). Tuina when applied by a skilled and knowledgeable practitioner, is a very effective form of therapy. Tuina uses the same theoretical and diagnostic principles that acupuncture does, however, the Qi in the meridians is stimulated strictly through the use of the hands or fingers through rubbing and pressing motions. No needles are used. Acupressure techniques are often used in conjunction with acupuncture or other TCM therapies.

There are many different ways in which tuina can stimulate the movement of Qi, each way specific to the type of therapeutic effect required (see Figures 12 and 13). Tuina is used mainly to treat musculoskeletal disorders and can be very relaxing, yet invigorating.

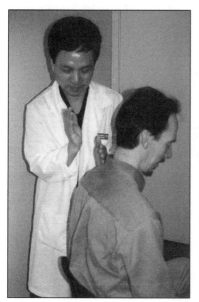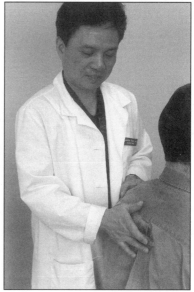

Figures 12 and 13: Dr. Jianfeng Yang Performing Tuina

MOXIBUSTION

Moxibustion is a common adjunctive technique that acupuncturists use. It treats disorders by applying heat at specific sites on or near the surface of the body. The heat generated during moxibustion is a very Yang form of Qi and activates the flow of Qi within the meridians. Moxibustion warms and nourishes the Qi of the body through the transferance of heat and can be used quite effectively for some underlying deficient conditions. The Yang Qi heat of moxibustion is also used specifically to dislodge coldness that may be trapped within the body. There are many ways to apply moxibustion to the skin surface, but two of the most common are the moxa pole (or stick) and rice grain moxa (see Figure 14).

These two methods use the same substance, a "punk" or "wool" obtained from the mugwort plant, *Artemesia vulgaris.* For the moxa

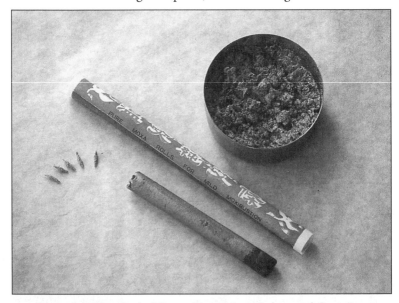

Figure 14: Rice Grain Moxa, Cigar Moxa Poles, and Container Holding Loose Moxa, or "Punk"

pole, the mugwort is compressed into cigar-like rolls. Use of the moxa pole is known as "indirect moxibustion." The pole is lit and held gently over the skin until the patient feels the area warming. In some instances the moxa pole is used at sites where acupuncture needles are already inserted. In this technique heat from the pole is transferred to the needle and carried deeper into the body.

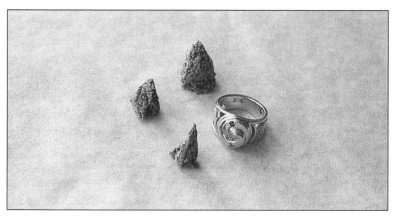

Figure 15: Moxa Cone Sizes Compaired with a Ring

Rice grain moxibustion and cone moxibustion are known as "direct moxibustion" because they use either small rice-sized moxa cones or larger moxa cones that are burned directly on the skin or ocassionally on a thin piece of ginger placed between the moxa cone and the skin. Larger moxa cones are generally 1/8" to 1/2" in size at the base. Most of the time the practitioner removes the burning cone

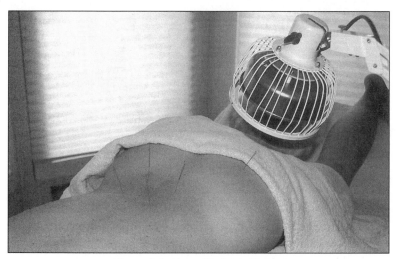

Figure 16: Use of Infrared Lamp

before it actually burns down to the skin surface, but not before the patient feels strong heat. Usually a practitioner uses between 5 and 9 cones of moxa at any given site. The number of cones or the length of time to use a moxa pole is determined by the requirements for an effective treatment (see Figure 15).

A recent addition to the method of application of external heat to the body is the use of infrared lamps (see Figure 16). These lamps are placed over the area to be warmed and turned on for 15 to 20 minutes. The heat they provide covers a more extensive area than either pole or cone moxibustion.

CUPPING

In cupping, a vacuum is created by lighting an alcohol swab and inserting it inside of a glass "cup" or jar, which is then quickly applied to the skin. This creates a suction that draws the skin slightly upward into the cup and helps to relieve congestion of Qi or Blood in the area where the cups are applied. Cups come in several sizes (see Figure 17). Traditionally, before the advent of modern glass-blowing, cups were made of bamboo. Even today, some practitioners still prefer using bamboo cups.

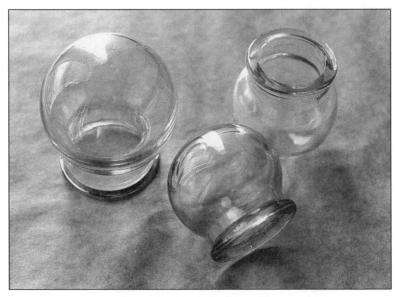

Figure 17: Variety of Cup Sizes

Cupping is often used in conjunction with acupuncture or moxibustion. Sometimes the cups are applied over an inserted needle, although most of the time they are used independently either before or after needle insertion. Cupping is used most frequently to treat sprains, sore muscles, and other types of musculoskeletal disorders. A special technique called "Running Cupping" is effective for back pain by applying the cup to oiled skin. The cup is then gently moved across the tissue.

Plum Blossom Needling

Plum Blossom needling, or Seven Star needling (see Figure 18), is a form of cutaneous needle therapy. In this technique needles are not inserted into the skin but used to stimulate the meridians by applying stimulation to the surface of the body. Both the Seven Star needle

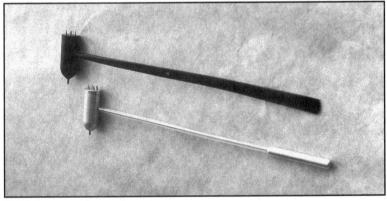

Figure 18: Plum Blossom and 7 Star Needles

and the Plum Blossom needle are composed of short stainless steel needles (seven or five respectively) in a bundle and attached to a handle. The needles are very short and have equal space between them.

In Plum Blossom needling the surface of the skin is tapped either heavily or lightly. Light tapping reddens the skin, and heavier tapping may cause slight bleeding. The area to be tapped may be a specific point or cover several points along a specific meridian. This technique stimulates the flow of both Qi and Blood to the area where the tapping is being applied. It is used for conditions of the nervous system and also skin disorders.

ELECTROACUPUNCTURE

Electroacupuncture applies a small electrical current to the inserted acupuncture needles. This type of therapy is relatively new in China and was developed during the 1930's. Traditionally, the application of a small current to the needles provided constant stimulation to the points and has been more often used to treat stubborn cases where the Qi is quite congested, such as hemiplegia or chronic musculoskeletal disorders. Recently, however, with the development of more technologically advanced electroacupuncture machines (see

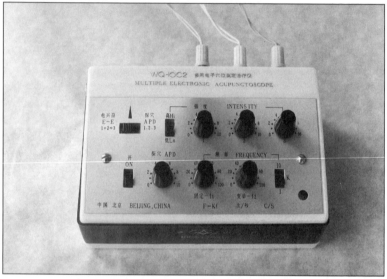

Figure 19: Electroacupuncture Machine

Figure 19), it has become more popular as a general mode of acupuncture therapy and anesthesia. The patient may or may not feel the electrical stimulation during the treatment. Electroacupuncture therapy usually lasts about 10 to 20 minutes per treatment.

CHINESE HERBAL MEDICINE

Chinese herbology is the other major branch of TCM. The premise of herbal medicine is that many plants and other materials, such as insects or minerals, have energetic properties that, when knowledgeably used, can have dramatic healing effects. The practice of Chinese herbology is truly an art, for the combining of herbs into just the right formula takes a great deal of skill and knowledge. There are literally hundreds of substances, mostly of plant origin, in the Chinese pharmacopoeia, and each substance has its own specific energetic properties.

Chinese herbal medicine uses the identical theoretic and diagnostic principles as does acupuncture. However, herbal medicine is traditionally used for more internal organ imbalances than acupuncture, which is used more predominantly in musculoskeletal disorders. The two therapeutic approaches of acupuncture and herbal medicine are quite complementary and are often used together in the same treatment. Each system affects the Qi of the body in specific ways. In many instances herbal remedies are used to supplement the body's Qi, and acupuncture is used to manipulate Qi, focusing it where it is needed. In essence, the general therapeutic approach to healing in Chinese medicine is that an individual must have Qi available in order to heal.

The art of Chinese herbal medicine lies in the development of the herbal formulas. Each formula contains many different herbal ingredients and each works synergistically with the others to bring about the therapeutic effect. When creating an herbal formula, each herb is given a place in an energetic hierarchy that uses names such as "chief," "deputy," "assistant," and " envoy." For example, the chief is the most important ingredient and holds the therapeutic focus of the entire formula. The deputy assists the chief in its duties by supplementing the focused approach or by treating secondary conditions. The assistant may foster the synergistic workings of the formula or assist in the prevention of possible toxic side effects, while the envoy may direct the formula to a specific body area or harmonize the actions of the other ingredients.

Herbal formulas generally have anywhere from five to twenty individual ingredients in them. Individual herbs are rarely, if ever, taken alone, for it is in combining the herbs that the true strength of herbal medicine lies. Each herb in a formula has a specific duty and energetic function. Some herbs draw energy downward in the body, for example, to treat gout, edema, or low back pain; while others cause energy to rise, for example, to treat headaches or upper body disorders. Many herbs bring Qi to the surface of the body, for example, to treat skin problems or to dispel flus or colds; whereas other herbs take Qi deeper to nourish or balance the internal organs. All herbs have attributes of flavor, for example, bitter, sweet or sour, and so on; temperature, for example, cold, neutral, hot, and so on; and specific meridians for which they have an affinity. For example, some herbs may enter the Spleen and Liver meridians, whereas others may enter the Lungs, Liver, and Kidneys, or any other combination of meridians. All these properties must be weighed when developing an herbal formula. It is no easy task and takes knowledge, patience, and a refined understanding of herbal and physiological energetics.

Herbal medicines can be prescribed in a number of ways. Two of the most common are prepared (or patent) herbs and raw herbs. Prepared herbs (see Figure 20) are usually classical Chinese herbal formulas in pill form and can be bought over the counter in herbal pharmacies. These formulas number in the hundreds and are used for specific health complaints.

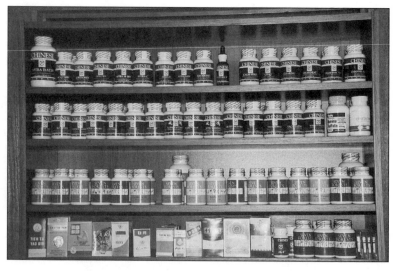

Figure 20: Selection of Patent Herbal Medicines

Prepared herbal medicines are manufactured in both China and the United States. The quality can vary a great deal from manufacturer to manufacturer, so it is best to consult a knowledgeable herbalist before choosing any prepared herbal formula.

Individual herbs in raw, unprepared form give the Chinese herbal pharmacy its customary earthy aroma. These herbal ingredients, mostly of plant origin, are usually stored in jars or large drawers and are used in decocting formulas for teas (see Figure 21). Measured portions of each ingredient in the herbal formula are selected, weighed and put together in a small bag. Each bag of ingredients is then added to boiling water, simmered, strained, then drunk. The method of preparation may be different for each formula, since some ingredients may require longer cooking time than others. There is usually enough for three or four cups of tea in each bag of ingredients.

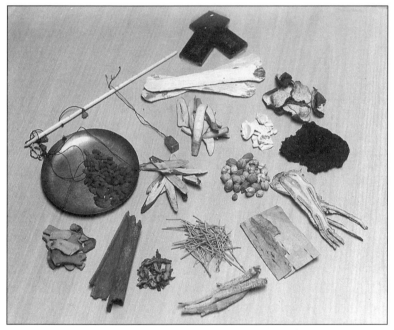

Figure 21: Sampling of Chinese Raw Herbs

If an herbalist does not have a raw herbal pharmacy, she may give a prescription to the patient to have it filled elsewhere. Some practitioners prefer to dispense prepared herbal medicines. The choice often depends on the therapeutic needs of the patient.

MEDICAL QI GONG

As we have seen, the manipulation of Qi for therapeutic purposes takes many forms. Perhaps least understood in the West is medical Qi Gong. This system enhances, clears, and focuses the flow of Qi through the body through specific body movements and visualizations. The therapeutic goals of medical Qi Gong are the same as those of other TCM modalities, however, in this therapy the practitioner

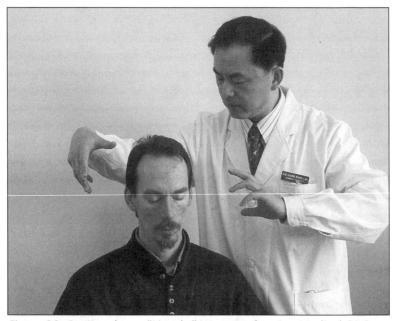

Figure 22: Dr. Xuezhong "Lincoln" Wang performing Medical Qi Gong

uses his or her hands to stimulate and manipulate the patient's Qi. The Qi Gong practitioner may not actually touch the patient, but manipulates the Qi of the patient from a short distance (see Figure 22).

In some instances the practitioner may teach specific medical Qi Gong techniques to a patient. This allows the patient to stimulate his or her own Qi on a regular basis without the need of the practitioner being present. Taiji is an example of a specific form of medical Qi Gong. In this practice individuals move their internal Qi in specific ways through physical movement and visualization. This helps to keep the Qi moving smoothly within the body, nourishing all tissues and keeping the muscles toned. Taiji can thus be seen as a form of medical Qi Gong that is preventative in nature.

Most hospitals in China have Qi Gong departments that work in concert with the acupuncture and herbal departments, as well as with the western medical departments. Medical Qi Gong is very subtle and takes a great deal of concentration and discipline to learn, but it can be very effective. Finding a qualified practitioner in the West can be difficult.

Case #7

Dan, a thin, middle-aged man, had been on high blood pressure medication for nearly eight years. These controlled his blood pressure, but the side effects caused him other concerns. He came to see me to find out if I could help him get off his blood pressure medication. I agreed, but only after I had spoken with his doctor and we agreed on a treatment strategy.

Dan was suffering from a condition where his Yin and Yang were out of balance. The Yang in his body was constantly rising up because the Yin was not holding it down. I treated Dan with acupuncture using points that helped to stabilize the rising energy in his body. At the same time I provided him with herbs that would help to nourish his deficient Yin. I also referred him to a medical Qi Gong practitioner who taught Dan how to redirect and nourish his own Qi through visualization and movement therapies.

Over the following weeks Dan had his blood pressure checked regularly by his physician as we slowly cut back on his medication. His doctor was quite surprised when after four months Dan was off his medications entirely and his blood pressure had stabilized at normal levels. Dan continues his Qi Gong practices daily and has resumed a normal healthy lifestyle.

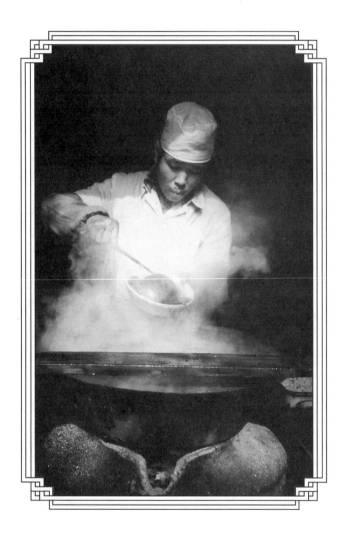

Chapter 4

Visiting a TCM Practitioner

Although the underlying principles of TCM are shared by all practitioners, the various techniques used vary from individual to individual. Many practitioners are very traditional and use only those techniques found in TCM. Other practitioners use techniques that have been developed in Japan or Korea or from research done here in the West. This chapter explores the experience of visiting a TCM practitioner, costs, and what to look for in a practitioner.

A Variety of Approaches to Treatment

The therapies encompassing TCM vary a great deal depending on the training and specialty of the individual practitioner. TCM has been modified by numerous cultural influences, and although these therapies still use acupuncture, the needling techniques vary. Sometimes the practitioner might also use a therapy that complements needling. For example, some practitioners may place small magnets on acupuncture points or meridians (Japanese). Others may use Korean Hand acupuncture, which employs only the microsystem of the hand to affect the overall Qi of the body. Other practitioners may specialize in specific diagnostic techniques such as Hara Diagnosis (Japanese), which focuses on palpating the abdomen. Still others may use ion-pumping cords (Japanese), a type of therapy that uses small cords connecting acupuncture needles inserted at different sites on the body. These are but a few of the many established techniques that practitioners in the United States, Canada, and Europe currently use to stimulate and move the Qi of the body. I expect the number and types of therapies to continue to expand as our knowledge and understanding of the dynamics of Qi continues to grow. With this said, however, we must still recognize that within the tradition of Chinese medicine, innumerable therapeutic approaches exist that reinforce, stimulate, and move the Qi. The modalities of acupuncture, herbal medicine, and tuina body therapy are a few of the most common that practitioners use in the United States.

VISITING A PRACTITIONER

Perceiving the entirety of an individual is a key to the effectiveness of any treatment. The practitioner and patient must work together to achieve therapeutic results. This can be an empowering experience for the patient, as well as for the practitioner. An important component of the therapeutic process is for the practitioner and patient to establish rapport. In relating to one another through communication based upon respect, trust, confidentiality and openness, the healing process begins.

Once mutual respect and trust are established, the next step is to gather information relating to the patient's condition. This is a seated interview that may take from 30 minutes to an hour. The practitioner gathers facts relating to the presenting problem, as well as a medical history and lifestyle information. This diagnostic interview uses the four examinations of Looking, Asking, Listening/Smelling, and Palpation, which were discussed in Chapter 2. The framework of the Eight Principles and/or the Five Elements is used to organize and prioritize all the information gathered. In developing a diagnosis, the practitioner considers all the components that contribute to the main problem, be they physical, emotional, mental, or spiritual, including the patient's demeanor, quality of voice, and all aspects of general appearance.

During the diagnostic interview the practitioner asks the patient questions, some of which may seem entirely unrelated to the problem at hand. The practitioner then checks the patient's tongue and pulses and, depending on the problem, may palpate specific sites on the patient's body. All these procedures are important in gathering the needed information to determine the correct diagnosis.

Based on the diagnosis, the practitioner chooses from a variety of therapeutic approaches to help realign the energies and reestablish balance of Qi within the patient. The most common of these modalities in the West is acupuncture. Many new patients naturally feel anxious when deciding to try acupuncture for the first time. The experience of receiving injection shots when we were young has left many of us with a healthy apprehension of needles. However, acupuncture needles are very different from the hypodermic needles used by western physicians and nurses. Acupuncture needles are very thin and fine. They are inserted either by hand or using a small guide tube. Nearly all new patients are pleasantly surprised and relieved when they first experience the insertion of an acupuncture needle. Anxiety diminishes rapidly. This is not to say that acupuncture needle insertion has no sensation associated with it, for depending on where the body is needled, the sensation can vary from none or slight to a moderate pricking feeling. Generally, the needles stay in for twenty or thirty minutes with the patient lying down. Sometimes the patient receives acupuncture sitting up, depending on where the needles need to be inserted. The practitioner may stimulate the needles periodically during this time in order to maintain the therapeutic effect. In some types of acupuncture therapy the treatment calls for leaving the needles in for only a few moments.

Acupuncture is generally very relaxing. During treatment it is not uncommon for patients to fall asleep. Often patients report a sense of well-being during the treatment that stays with them throughout the day. Receiving acupuncture gives a person time to rest and allows the forces of Qi stimulated by the treatment to help reestablish harmony to the mind, body, and spirit.

Sometimes physical conditions require more than just one type of therapeutic intervention. In these instances a practitioner may also use moxibustion, cupping, or tuina, or suggest specific herbal formulas to help enhance the therapeutic effects. Sometimes counseling or major lifestyle changes are also suggested adjuncts to the therapies of TCM.

Counseling is recommended when a strong emotional or spiritual component may be an underlying factor contributing to a physical illness. It should be remembered that a longstanding imbalance in the emotions or mind can create imbalances in the body. To resolve illness may require not only work to balance the Qi of the physical body, but also work geared to balance the Qi that orchestrates the mind and emotions. The number of treatments an individual requires depends on the condition that brought him or her to the practitioner in the first place. In TCM an old adage states, "For each year an imbalance has occurred, it will take one month of treatment." So, if an individual has had chronic back pain for six years, this may require a few months of acupuncture therapy.

More acute conditions, such as colds and flus or recent sprains or strains, may be resolved relatively quickly with only a few treatments. In many instances an individual presents with internal deficiencies of Qi that need to be nourished and restored before the individual has enough energy to help completely heal or repair their body.

There are many facets to illness and all must be weighed when determining the correct treatment strategy and the number of treatments required to resolve a condition.

Most conditions respond well. Some, due to the chronicity or severity of the condition, may respond very little or not at all. Another primary factor in the resolution of many disorders is the willingness of the patient to cooperate with the treatment approach. For example, if a patient has a chronic cough that disrupts sleep, but is unwilling to stop smoking, there is little a practitioner can do to help resolve the cough.

Cost

TCM is very cost-effective and is much less expensive than conventional medicine. The cost of visiting a TCM practitioner varies for different regions of the country. The average fee for a first appointment generally ranges from $45 to $80 and usually takes about one and a half hours. Return appointments generally range from about $35 to $55 for an hour. A monthly supply of herbs usually cost $6 to $18 per bottle for patent medicines and $25 to $50 for raw herbal formulas. Raw herbal formulas are more tailored to the patient's needs and thus may have more on an immediate therapeutic impact than patent medicines. This is why the large difference in price between raw and herbal formulas. Some insurance companies cover TCM therapies such as acupuncture. An insurance company representative can let you know if this is the case. Insurance coverage for TCM is changing rapidly and major insurance companies are now starting to cover many specific conditions.

FINDING A PRACTITIONER

Choosing a competent TCM practitioner is an important part of achieving good therapeutic results. There are many organizations in the United States that have listings of trained and qualified practitioners throughout the country (see Appendix C). Also, check to see if there is a school of Oriental Medicine near you. Schools have listings of their graduates and are a good referral source. Many states where TCM is licensed have professional organizations. Check your phone book. Most professional state organizations keep an updated referral list of qualified practitioners.

Check to see if the TCM practitioner is certified, licensed, or registered. Not only do the designations vary from state to state, but the requirements for these various designations vary as well. It is best to check with each state individually to determine how they define these designations. Choose a practitioner who can practice legally in your state.

It is also important to find out where the practitioner studied and for how long (see Appendix D for further information on education, training, and certification). Also, check to see if the illness that you are seeking help for is treatable by TCM (see Appendix B for a list of diseases treated by TCM). Other questions to consider are: Does the practitioner use disposable needles? What are the costs for each treatment? How long are the first office appointment and follow-up visits? How long has the practitioner been in practice? Has the practitioner had any complaints registered against him or her with the state? These are a few of the questions that will assist you in finding a well-trained, legal, and experienced TCM practitioner.

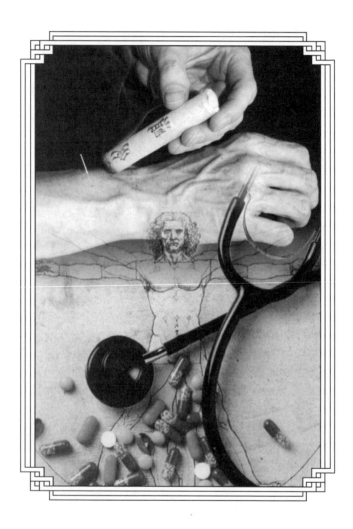

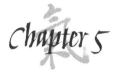

Chapter 5

THE FUTURE:
WORLD MEDICINE

The face of medicine is changing. Western medicine is exploring new frontiers in psychology and bioenergetics, and the East is discovering the power of pharmaceuticals and the coronary bypass. There is a peculiar beauty to this balance and, hopefully, some significant benefits to humanity. This chapter explores the possibilites of the medicine of tomorrow.

PERSONAL PERSPECTIVES

Recently, a growing number of "Body-Mind-Spirit" health-related seminars are being presented throughout the United States. The importance of this more-than-mechanistic perspective was not given much medical credence in the West until recently. The influences on the body of subtle energies such as electromagnetism, microwaves, thoughts, emotions, prayer, sun spots, weather, and so on, are now being investigated. The premise is that we can greatly influence the well-being of our physical bodies through our thoughts and emotions. I believe the integration of the Body-Mind-Spirit paradigm with western medical thinking is primarily due to the influences of eastern philosophy and eastern medicine over the last 30 years. This type of thinking is a fundamental premise within TCM.

Oriental medicines (Chinese, Japanese, Korean, East Indian, etc.) have incorporated the concepts of energetic medicine for thousands of years. Out of these ancient systems developed the concept of Qi (Ki, Prana), the vital subtle force that impels all life forms. Ancient healers were quite advanced in their understanding of how energy influences the body, and this knowledge continues to be the foundation on which TCM is based.

Western medicine has now begun to incorporate the concepts of the integrated Body-Mind-Spirit system that TCM has traditionally used. TCM has long stood as an enigma for western medicine, for it forces the issue on subtle energetic influences that affect the body. It forces the western mind to look beyond the single-focused, mechanistic approach to health care and to open to new possibilities. Acupuncture has especially piqued the interest of the scientific community. Researchers, both within Asia and the West, are beginning to take a closer look at the efficacy of acupuncture and its possible mechanisms of action. Physicists are concluding that the more subtle forces of Qi may be at work more than were previously thought. The results of this research, along with the demands of the public, have led to the development of this "new" western science—Energy Medicine.

Although eastern and western perspectives on Energy Medicine may appear quite different, they actually share many similarities. These schools of thought discuss many of the same concepts and healing techniques but use different language. It is as though each is focusing on different aspects of the same system. I believe that this is more a cultural phenomenon and largely a matter of semantics and terminology. Such cultural bias can lead to the false assumption that these are distinct and different energetic systems. However, the universal energy of Qi has innumerable forms and can be described in myriad ways, and these varying descriptions do not make it "different." As these cultural perspectives continue to influence one another, they will eventually evolve into a more dynamic global form of Energy Medicine, one in which the language and concepts are synchronous.

The influences of energy on the well-being of all of us are significant. It matters not whether the energy is cloaked in the TCM framework of "Qi" or the western understanding of electrons, protons, or neutrons. It is the same energy.

The following examples show some of the similarities of eastern and western concepts and approaches to Energy Medicine.

—A western therapy may encourage a cancer patient to mentally visualize internal forces destroying the cancer cells. Medical Qi Gong may use the same approach, teaching the patient the power of mind necessary to overcome and dissolve cancerous tissues.

—The power of forgiveness has become an important component for healing. Forgiveness allows for emotional release by dispelling an unhealthy emotional/mental environment in which diseases can gain a foothold. In TCM, balancing the organ systems that influence the emotions is a major component of preventative medicine. In TCM, it is said that constraint of emotions (being unforgiving) often leads to disease.

—In both eastern and western cultures the health benefits of meditation have been known for years. Meditation calms the mind and helps to establish a rapport with the higher spiritual dimensions within. The discipline of meditation can be a powerful integrative factor for establishing a sense of spiritual well being, emotional equanimity, and physical health.

—Environmental and electromagnetic pollution are being acknowledged as having potentially dangerous influences on our state of health. Some of these external energetic factors have been implicated in immune system disorders. In TCM, the concept of " External Evils" is well known. These "evils" can be represented as everything from the common cold virus to electromagnetic and chemical sensitivities. TCM's approach to healing these conditions is to strengthen the body to ward off negative invading forces.

—Some groups within the Energy Medicine movement speak of the major chakras, or seven energy centers, which influence the different energetic levels of our body, mind, emotions, and spirit. The chakra system has been a part of the East Indian energy system for thousands of years. It has only recently been incorporated into some western healing methods.

—Western minds are beginning to realize that specific living and working environments may strongly influence how we think, feel, and respond physiologically. The color of a room or the placement of a desk, plant, or mirror can have subtle energetic consequences for those residing in that environment. Feng Shui (fung shway), the ancient Chinese "art of placement" (or literally "the way of wind and water") has been employed by Asian cultures for centuries to create optimal energetic environments for a healthy state of being. In Feng

Shui it is the balance of Yin and Yang that is being cultivated.

My vision for the future is that the reciprocal influences of the East and West—right brain/left brain, Yin/Yang—will of necessity and by demand create a wholistic World Medicine. This World Medicine will be rooted in the traditions of the multidimensionality of human beings honoring intuition as a major healing tool. It will incorporate the understanding that the emotions, mind, and spirit are vital components in both our well-being and disease. Medicine will walk hand in hand with the individual, encouraging and empowering responsible self-health care. It will focus on assisting healing the whole being, not just the physical body. World Medicine will incorporate energetic systems and education to help bring about the expansion of consciousness, intuition, compassion, longevity and optimal health.

Appendix A

A Brief History of Traditional Chinese Medicine

This very brief summary of some of the more important events and people that shaped the development of Chinese medical history also touches upon the expansion of TCM into Europe and the United States. Many thousands of texts have been written regarding Chinese medicine over the centuries. Listed below are a few of the most significant of these books and their authors.

Prehistoric Period

- Roots of Shamanic healing: W*u* -" women who can bring down spirits". Shamans were mostly women and the primary healer/ priests during this time period. The shaman would go into trance during ritual healing. The shamanic repertoire consisted of exorcism, divination, prophecy, fertility rites, and healing. Wu used bells, drums, knives, medicines, and chants to assist them in their work. In exorcism the Wu used self-torture, often inflicting wounds on herself as well as the patient. Treatment could be fatal to both.

Yangshao Culture 5000 B.C.

- Shen Nong, the forefather of Chinese medicine and "God of Husbandry," is said to have taught the ancient people how to raise crops and domestic animals as well as how to identify medicinal plants.
- Stone (*bian*) needles used to apply pressure to sore points on the body, not for piercing the skin.

Langshan Culture 2500 B.C.

- Legendary figure Huang Di, or the Yellow Emperor, is said to have existed. He is considered to be the ancestor of the Chinese race and the author of the ancient medical text *The Yellow Emperor's Classic of Internal Medicine*.
- Mythological figure Fu Xi, the legendary author of the *I Ching*, or *Book of Changes*. This book of divination beautifully expounds upon the principles of Yin and Yang. Fu Xi is said to have invented the calendar and musical instruments as well as having taught the ancient Chinese people hunting and fishing.

Three Rulers and Five Emperors 2852 - 2205 B.C.

Xia Dynasty 2205 - 1766 B.C.

B.C.Shang Dynasty 1766 - 1122 B.C.

- First known written medical records on tortoise shell and animal bones. Archeological findings also include crude bone and stone acupuncture needles (*bian*).

Zhou Dynasty 1122 - 256 B.C.

Warring States Period 403 - 221 B.C.

- *Yellow Emperor's Classic of Internal Medicine* (*Huang Di Neijing*) compiled from medical experience and theoretical knowledge up to this time.
- *The Classic of Difficulties* (*Nanjing*) compiled. Addresses difficult passages from the *Yellow Emperor's Classic of Internal Medicine*.
- Metal needles start being used with the development of metallurgy. First needles were bronze.
- Chinese herbal formulas written on wooden slips.

Qin Dynasty 221- 206 B.C.

Han Dynasty 206 B.C. - A.D. 220

- *Treatise on Febrile Diseases* (*Shang Han Za Bing Lun*) authored by Zhang Zhongjing. Today in China it is still considered one of the primary texts on herbal medicine.
- Basics of TCM theory and practice firmly in place.
- Hua Tou, China's first surgeon, (110 - 207).

Three Kingdoms 220 - 280

- Wang Suho arranged the *Shang Han Za Bing Lun* into 2 texts: *Treatise on Febrile Diseases* (*Shang Han Lun*) and the *Summaries of Household Remedies* (*Jin Gui Yao Lue*)
- *The Book of Acupuncture Fundamentals* (*Jia Yi Jing*) attributed to Huangfu Mi.

Western Jin 265 - 316

- *Classic of Acupuncture and Moxibustion* (*Zhenjiu Jiayijing*) by Huangfu Mi.
- *Emergency Prescriptions to Keep Up One's Sleeves* (*Zhouhou Beiji Fang*) attributed to Ge Hong.

Southern and Northern Dynasties 317 - 589
- Tao Hongjing compiled the *Divine Husbandman's Classic of the Materia Medica* (*Shen Nong Ben Cao Jing*) which was originally attributed to the "Divine Husbandman", Shen Nong.

Sui Dynasty 589 - 618
- Sun Simiao wrote *Thousand Golden Prescriptions for Medical Emergencies* (*Bei Ji Qian Jin Yao Fang*) and the *Golden Supplementary Prescriptions* (*Qian Jin Yi Fang*).
- Foundation of the Imperial Medical College with acupuncture as a unit in the medical department.

Tang Dynasty 618 - 907
- Establishment of the Imperial Academy of Medicine with four departments: internal medicine, acupuncture, massage and sorcery.

Five Dynasties and Ten Kingdoms 907 - 960

Song Dynasty 960 - 1279
- Illustrated Manual on Points for Acupuncture and Moxibustion Shown on a Bronze Figure (*Tongren Shuxue Zhenjiu Tujing*) by Wang Weiyi.
- 2 nearly life-sized bronze statues created depicting the meridians and points of acupuncture.
- *Meridian Points and Moxibustion Techniques* (*Gao Huang Yu*) by Chuang Cao.
- Foundation of an official agency to supply and dispense herbal medicine.

Yuan Dynasty 1279 - 1368
- *The Divine Response Classic* (*Shen Ying Jing*) written by Chen Hui. This book contained rhymes accompanied by illustrations for over 119 acupuncture points.
- Wang Guorui composed *The Jade Dragon Classic of the Efficacious Acupuncture and Moxibustion of Bian Que* (*Bian Que Shenying Zhenjiu Yulong Jin*). This book of rhymes contained 120 acupuncture points.

Ming Dynasty 1368 - 1644
- 3 more bronze statues cast: a man, woman, and child, all depicting the meridians and points of acupuncture.

- *On Pulse Diagnosis* (*Bin Hu Mai Xue*) by Li Shizhen. This book described the 27 pulse types in verse. *Complete Collection of Acupuncture and Moxibustion* (*Zhenjiu Daquan*) written by Xu Feng.
- Wang Ji wrote *Questions and Answers About Acupuncture and Moxibustion* (*Zhenjiu Wendui*).
- Appearance of moxa rolls towards the end of the 14 century.

Qing Dynasty 1644 - 1911

- Chinese medicine spreads to Europe with *Secrets de la Medicine des Chinois* published in France in 1671. Author was anonymous. Many publications followed over the next few years.
- *Golden Mirror of Medicine*: an encyclopedia of medicine compiled in 1742.

Republic of China 1911 - 1949

- Cheng Dan-an (1899 - 1957) establishes the Chinese Acupuncture Research Society, founded the Chinese Acupuncture Specialty School, and ran an acupuncture correspondence school.
- TCM prohibited in 1929.

Peoples' Republic of China 1949 - present

- Renaisssance of TCM.
- Research (1950's) on the use of acupuncture anesthesia begins in the mid-1950's.
- The development of ear acupuncture is expanded in China from knowledge received from Europe.
- President Richard Nixon visits China in 1971. This initiates the growth of TCM in the United States.
- Between 1972 - 75, two acupuncture journals started in the United States; currently over 33 colleges of acupuncture and Oriental Medicine that are accredited or candidates for accreditation in the U.S.; 35 states license TCM; establishment of an accreditation agency to accredit TCM schools; national exam for certification established; and the creation of two national professional organizations (see Appendix C).

Appendix B

World Health Organization's List of Diseases Helped with Traditional Chinese Medicine

The World Health Organization (WHO) recognizes the ability of acupuncture and Oriental medicine to treat over 43 commonly encountered clinical disorders. In the United States, acupuncture is most commonly known for the treatment of pain and drug detoxification. Among the most common disorders for treatment recognized by WHO are:

Alcohol dependence	High Blood Pressure
Allergies/Asthma	Immune system deficiency
Anxiety/Depression	Infertility
Arthritis/Joint problems	Insomnia
Back pain	Knee pain
Bladder/Kidney problems	Fibromyocitis
Carpal tunnel syndrome	Neck pain/Stiffness
Childhood illness	Numbness/Poor circulation
Colds/Flu/Cough/Bronchitis	Premenstrual syndrome
Constipation/Diarrhea	Sciatica
Dizziness	Sexual dysfunction/Impotence
Drug Addiction/Smoking	Shoulder pain
Eye, ear, nose and throat disorders	Skin problems
Fatigue	Sports injuries
Gynecological disorders	Stress/Tension
Headache/Migraine	Tendinitis
Heart problems/Palpitations	TMJ/Jaw pain
Herpes	Weight gain or loss

Appendix C

National Organizations

There are a number of national organizations associated with Oriental medicine. Below is a partial list of the most important organizations and their roles in Oriental medical education and the profession.

COUNCIL OF COLLEGES OF ACUPUNCTURE
AND ORIENTAL MEDICINE (CCAOM)
1010 WAYNE AVE., #1270, SILVER SPRING, MD 20910
(301) 608-9175   FAX (301) 608-9576

The Council of Colleges was formed in 1982 for the purpose of advancing the status of acupuncture and Oriental medicine in the United States. The Council has developed academic and clinical guidelines and core curriculum requirements for master's level programs in acupuncture as well as acupuncture and Oriental medicine.

On-going work of the Council includes programs in faculty and administrative development; support of research, translation and other academic work in Oriental medicine; guidelines in institutional development for member colleges and support of member and non-member colleges in their work towards accreditation. As of 1997 there are 33 members of the Council.

ACCREDITATION COMMISSION FOR
ACUPUNCTURE AND ORIENTAL MEDICINE (ACAOM)
1010 WAYNE AVE., #1270, SILVER SPRING, MD 20910
(301) 608-9175   FAX (301) 608-9576
FORMERLY NATIONAL ACCREDITATION COMMISSION FOR
SCHOOLS AND COLLEGES OF ACUPUNCTURE AND ORIENTAL
MEDICINE (NACSCAOM)

The Accreditation Commission was established in June, 1982 by the Council of Colleges of Acupuncture and Oriental Medicine. The Commission acts as an independent body to evaluate first professional master's degree and first professional master's level certificate and diploma programs in both acupuncture and Oriental medicine with concentrations in both acupuncture and herbal therapy for a level of performance, integrity and quality that entitles them to the

confidence of the educational community and the public they serve.
The Commission establishes accreditation criteria, arranges site visits, evaluates those programs that desire accredited status and publicly designates those programs that meet the criteria. The accrediting process requires each program to examine goals, activities and outcomes; to consider the criticism and suggestions of a visiting team; to determine internal procedures for action on recommendations from the Commission; and to maintain continuous self-study and improvement mechanisms.

The Commission is recognized by the U.S. Department of Education and the Council for Higher Education Accreditation and is a charter member of the Association of Specialized and Professional Accreditors.

NATIONAL COMMISSION FOR THE CERTIFICATION OF ACUPUNCTURE AND ORIENTAL MEDICINE (NCCAOM)
1424 16TH STREET N.W., SUITE 501
WASHINGTON D.C. 20036
(202) 232-1404   FAX (202) 462-6157
FORMERLY NATIONAL COMMISSION FOR THE CERTIFICATION OF ACUPUNCTURISTS (NCCA)

The NCCAOM was established by the profession in 1982 to develop and implement nationally recognized standards of competence for the practice of acupuncture and Oriental medicine. Since its inception, the NCCAOM has certified over six thousand Diplomates of Acupuncture and is used as the basis for licensure in 90% of the states which have established standards of practice for acupuncture. The NCCAOM administers the national Board examinations for the profession of acupuncture and Oriental medicine. These exams are both written and practical and test medical proficiency in the theory, diagnosis, treatment, referral, and ethics of the Oriental medicine profession.

Certification in acupuncture is based on a candidate's ability to meet eligibility standards of education and/or experience; passage of the comprehensive written and practical examinations; successful completion of an NCCAOM approved Clean Needle Technique Course and committment to the professional code of ethics.

The NCCAOM is a member of the National Organization of Competency Assurance and certified by the National Commission for Certifying Agents, the agency with the highest voluntary standards of certifying agencies in the United States.

NATIONAL ACUPUNCTURE AND
ORIENTAL MEDICINE ALLIANCE (NAOMA)
14637 STARR ROAD S.E., OLALLA, WA 98359
(253) 851-6896   FAX (253) 851-6883

The National Alliance is one of two national professional membership associations. It was founded in 1993 to represent the diversity of practitioners of acupuncture and Oriental medicine in the United States.

AMERICAN ASSOCIATION OF
ORIENTAL MEDICINE (AAOM)
433 FRONT STREET, CATASAUQUA, PA 18032
(610) 266-1433   FAX (610) 264-2768

The AAOM is the other professional membership organization in the United States. It was established in 1982 and is a specialty membership organization representing one segment and philosophy within the profession.

Appendix D

Education and Scope of Practice

Within the United States, Oriental medical education has advanced greatly within the last twenty-five years. Currently there are over thirty accredited schools of acupuncture and Oriental medicine in America. These schools have been granted accreditation by the Accreditation Commission for Acupuncture and Oriental Medicine (ACAOM). ACAOM is recognized by the U.S. Department of Education and the Council of Higher Education Accreditation.

Schools of Oriental medicine are currently divided into two groups: those which offer education in acupuncture only and those which offer education in acupuncture and Chinese herbology. All accredited schools offer degrees or diplomas at the Masters level of education. Admission into these schools requires a minimum of two years of baccalaureate education. Some schools require three years, others require a full four year baccalaureate degree. The titles of the masters degrees offered vary from school to school and can range from a Master of Acupuncture (M.Ac.) to a Master of Traditional Chinese Medicine (M.T.C.M.). Other titles include: Master of Science (M.S.), Master of Acupuncture and Oriental Medicine (M.A.O.M.), Master of Science of Acupuncture and Oriental Medicine (M.S.A.O.M.), Master of Traditional Oriental Medicine (M.T.O.M.), etc.

The educational guidelines of accedited schools are established by CCAOM and are evaluated by ACAOM. Educational guidelines include studies in Oriental medical history, theory and techniques, diagnostic principles, western biomedical concepts, medical referral, hygiene, ethics and hundreds of hours of clinical observation and internship under the supervision of licensed acupuncturists and herbalists. Students are taught how to interface with western medicine and are knowledgable of when referral to a western medical practitioner is appropriate.

In most states in order to become licensed the practitioner must have graduated from a school approved by the licensing agency and must have passed a national examination which consists of both written and practical portions. Most states also have avenues for licensure for individuals who have graduated from credible foreign schools of Oriental medicine, such as those in China, Korea, or Japan.

The licensing laws and scope of practice of Oriental medicine varies widely from state to state. In most states a practitioner is able to work independently, usually offering services through private clinics or group practices. In other states the practitioner must work under the supervision of a western physician, and still in others there are no laws governing the practice of Oriental medicine at all. For specific information on each state see "Acupuncture and Oriental Medicine State Laws" published by the National Acupuncture Foundation. It may be ordered through Bookmasters, (800) 247-6553.

The education, licensing, and scope of practice of Oriental medical practitioners has gained a strong foothold in this country. This is due primarily to its clinical efficacy and support by those who have experienced its therapeutic results.

Appendix E

Synopsis of Safety Record
of Acupuncture and Oriental Medicine

Due to the growing demand for acupuncture and Oriental medical services, regulators throughout the United States are faced with setting standards to protect the public. One of the first questions which surfaces is the risk of harm involving Oriental medicine, especially acupuncture. The evidence shows that, when performed by trained individuals, acupuncture is an extremely safe procedure and has a remarkably low record of accidents.

The synopsis of the Safety Record of Acupuncture, available from the National Acupuncture Foundation, (202) 332-5794, reflects reports in the medical literature in English from 1958 to 1995 from the United States, West Germany, England, Israel, Ireland, Australia, Japan, China, Spain, Belgium and Switzerland. This document shows a remarkable safety record for acupuncture around the world.

Regarding the risk of injury to internal organs, acupuncturists are trained in exact needle placement, angle and depth of insertion. This results in extremely low risk of injury when acupuncture is performed by a competent individual. This is demonstrated by the following:

In China and Japan, both of which have excellent training programs for acupuncturists and thousands of treatments annually, only ten injuries to internal organs have been reported since 1972.

No injuries have been reported in Korea. In the United States, only ten incidents of injury have been reported since 1965.

Of the ten cases in the United States, one was noted as a "one-in- a-million" complication, another as a bizarre set of circumstances involving self-inflicted injury by an untrained individual.

Of the reports from the United States, only one specified that the treatment had been performed by a licensed or certified acupuncturist and that individual was licensed without examination or standards of competency.

In the reports from other Western countries, in most of which only MD's may practice acupuncture, it was unclear who had performed the treatment.

GLOSSARY OF TERMS

Acupressure

Uses the same underlying principles of TCM but treatment is applied by pressure and massage instead of the use of needles.

Acupuncture

TCM healing therapy which inserts fine needles into specific points on the body in order to reestablish balance or unblock the flow of energy in the body.

Acupuncture Points

Specific sites on the body where the energy from within the body comes to the surface and can be adjusted through the use of acupuncture or acupressure.

Acute

A disorder of short duration.

Body Fluids

The fluids of the body which nourish and moisten, lubricate, surround and protect various tissues.

Chakra

A subtle energy center of the body for giving and receiving life force.

Channels

Subtle energy pathways which carry the flow of Qi on the surface of the body as well as deep within the body; also called meridians.

Chronic

A disorder which has persisted for a long time.

Cupping

A treatment technique whereby suction is applied to the skin surface using small jars in which a vacuum is created.

Damp

One of the climatic "Six Evils" in TCM which can invade the body leading to sluggishness, sensations of heaviness in the body, tiredness and general lassitude.

Decoction

A raw herbal preparation with measured quantities of specific herbs that are boiled in water together to make a tea for drinking.

Deficient Condition
Any disorder that is the result of the body's inability to maintain balance through weakened functioning of the internal organs.

De Qi
The sensation of tingling or heaviness felt by the patient when the Qi in the meridians is accessed upon insertion of an acupuncture needle.

Diagnosis
The process of deciding the nature of a diseased condition by examination of the symptoms.

Disharmony
A lack of balance and harmony in the body often resulting in disease.

Eight Principles
The system of organizing diagnostic information in TCM according to the paired principles of Yin/Yang; Interior/Exterior; Cold/Hot; and Deficiency/Excess.

Excess Condition
A state in which accumulation occurs within the body, either from an imbalance of the organ system or from an invasion from outside the body by a pathogenic factor.

External
Any factor which influences the body, mind or spirit from outside.

Feng Shui
In Chinese culture, the "Art of Placement" which analyzes the energy patterns of the external environment in relation to their effects on living organisms.

Five Elements
The system of organizing TCM principles based on observations of the natural world; the Five Elements are wood, fire, earth, metal and water.

Fu
The six hollow Yang organs of the body; they are the stomach, small intestine, large intestine, urinary bladder, gall bladder and the triple warmer.

Gu Qi
The Qi extracted from the foods that we eat; also called Food Qi.

Internal
Refers to aspects of disharmony that arise from within the body.

Jing
The vital essence stored in the Kidneys which is the source of life, growth and development.

Luo
The system of connecting channels which carry Qi between the major meridians.

Medical Qi Gong
A TCM modality that enhances, clears and focuses the flow of Qi through the body through specific movements and visualizations.

Meridians
The channels through which Qi flows throughout the body; there are many types of meridians, the most common being the 12 Primary meridians on which the majority of acupuncture points are located.

Modality
The employment of a specific therapeutic agent; in TCM the main modalities include acupuncture, acupressure, herbalism, and medical Qi Gong.

Moxa
Dried mugwort, *Artemisia vulgaris*, which is burned on inserted acupuncture needles, rolled into a stick and then burned close to the skin, or made into small cones and burned directly on the skin; also see moxibustion.

Moxibustion
The therapeutic treatment involving the burning of moxa which produces heat to warm the body and activate the Qi.

Palpation
The process of examination with the hands.

Pathogenic
Causing or producing disharmony or disease.

Postnatal Qi
Qi which is created from the foods we eat and the air we breathe; also referred to as Post-Heaven Qi.

Prenatal Qi

Qi which we receive from our parents in the form of heredity; also referred to as Pre-Heaven Qi.

Qi

The Chinese term for vital energy; in TCM it is the life force which is fundamental to the creation and functioning of all aspects of life; it travels throughout the body in the meridians.

Sedation

In TCM the process of dispersing an accumulation of Qi in the body.

Shen

The most rarified form of Qi in TCM which corresponds to Mind or Spirit.

Tonification

The process of strengthening the body, especially the elements of Qi and Blood.

Triple Warmer

The Triple Heater/Burner/Energizer, San Jiao; the energy which integrates and unifies the Qi of the three cavities of the body: the thoracic, abdominal and pelvic.

Wei Qi

The Qi which flows just beneath the skin and protects the body from external pathogenic influences; also called Protective Qi.

Yang

One pole, or aspect, of the dualistic nature of reality; it represents the more active, moving, bright and functional aspects.

Yin

One pole, or aspect, of the dualistic nature of reality; it represents the quiescent, reflective, darker and material aspects.

Ying Qi

The aspect of Qi which nurtures the body and is activated with the insertion of an acupuncture needle; also called Nutritive Qi.

Yuan Qi

The active form of Jing; the foundation of all the Yin and Yang energies of the body; also called Source Qi.

Zang

The six solid Yin organs of the body; they are the lungs, heart, liver, spleen, kidney and pericardium.

Zang Fu

The TCM term which denotes the functional activities of the twelve Yin and Yang organ systems in the body.

References

Capra, Fritjof. *The Tao of Physics.* New York: Bantam Books, 1975.

Kaptchuk, Ted J. *The Web That Has No Weaver: Understanding Chinese Medicine.* New York: Congdon & Weed, 1983.

Gerber, Richard. *Vibrational Medicine: New Choices for Healing Ourselves.* Santa Fe: Bear & Company, 1988.

Govert, Johndennis. *Feng Shui: Art and Harmony of Placement.* Phoenix: Daikakuji Publications, 1993.

Hiep, Nguyen Duc. *The Dictionary of Acupuncture and Moxibustion: A Practical Guide to Traditional Chinese Medicine.* Rochester: Thorsons Publishers Inc., 1987.

Lade, Arnie. *Acupuncture Points, Images & Functions.* Seattle: Eastland Press, 1989.

Larre, Claude, and Elisabeth Rochat de la Vallee. *The Seven Emotions: Psychology and Health in Ancient China.* Cambridge, U.K.: Monkey Press, 1996.

Maciocia, Giovanni. *The Foundations of Chinese Medicine: A Comprehensive Text for Acupuncturists and Herbalists.* New York: Churchill Livingstone, 1989.

Millenson, J.R. *Mind Matters: Psychological Medicine in Holistic Practice.* Seattle: Eastland Press, 1995.

Myss, Caroline M. *Anatomy of the Spirit.* New York: Harmony Books, 1996.

Ross, Jeremy. *Zang Fu: The Organ Systems of Traditional Chinese Medicine.* Edinburgh: Churchill Livingstone, 1984.

Shealy, C. Norman, and Caroline M. Myss. *The Creation of Health.* Walpole, N.H.: Stillpoint Publishing, 1993.

Unschuld, Paul U. *Medicine in China: A History of Ideas.* University of California Press, 1985.

Wilhelm, Richard. *The I Ching or Book of Changes.* Translated by Cary F. Baynes. New York: Bollingen Foundation, 1950.

INDEX